The Tales & Tails of a
Yorkshire Vet

The Tales & Tails of a Yorkshire Vet

ALL IN A DAY'S WORK FOR
PETER WRIGHT

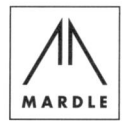

MARDLE

Published in 2023 by Mardle Books
15 Church Road
London, SW13 9HE
www.mardlebooks.com

Text © 2023 Peter Wright

ISBN 9781914451782
eBook ISBN 9781837700455

All rights reserved. No part of this publication may be reproduced in any form or by any means — electronic, mechanical, photocopying, recording, or otherwise — or stored in any retrieval system of any nature without prior written permission from the copyright holders. Peter Wright has asserted his moral right to be identified as the author of this work in accordance with the Copyright, Designs and Patents Act of 1988.

Photographs used with permission of Daisybeck Studios/Motion Content Group and Barry Marsden Photography.

A CIP catalogue record for this book is available from the British Library.

Typeset by Danny Lyle

Printed in the UK
10 9 8 7 6 5 4 3 2 1

MIX
Paper from responsible sources
FSC
www.fsc.org
FSC® C018072

To the many fans and contributors of
The Yorkshire Vet. This is for you.

Contents

1 Early animals	1
2 Wet behind the ears	14
3 Thirsk for knowledge	31
4 Risky business	45
5 Sometimes all you can do is laugh	60
6 Sad cases	77
7 Miracles do happen	88
8 Strange cases	104
9 Cock and bull stories	122
10 'Ow do, pet?	136
11 My life in pets	153
12 Yorkshire, through and through	177
13 Green energy	191
14 Donkeys, ducks and wildlife	203
15 Goodbye Skeldale	217
16 Hello Grace Lane	226
Acknowledgements	243

1

Early animals

Norman Knowles was a Wesleyan Methodist and as such he did not drink and he did not use profanities.

'By Jove,' was as strong an exclamation as you were likely to hear from him. He was a genial, God-fearing man who would do anything for anyone and ran the 180-acre Manor Farm, not far from the North Yorkshire market town of Thirsk where I grew up and still live. His only vice was smoking. You would rarely see him without a cigarette hanging from his lips. It would bob up and down when he talked and the ash would drop from it when it got too long, because once he'd started a smoke, Norman rarely removed it from his mouth.

He was a lovely man and had a good sense of humour. His wife, Joan, who died recently at the age of over a 100, was a fervent churchgoer who hardly missed a Sunday service. Norman enjoyed cooking, which was unusual for a man at the time. Joan would go to church on Sunday, while Norman stayed at home.

My grandfather, Fred, worked on Norman's farm as a farm manager. Previously, he'd tried to work on his in-laws' farm but couldn't get on with them so he left and went to work for Norman, as did my dad, Ken, who worked as a labourer there too for a time. They were treated as friends, not employees. Norman wasn't one to work his fingers to the bone. He appeared to have many aunts whom he would regularly take to the seaside or for afternoon tea.

Norman had a dog, a black-and-white border collie named Pip. Pip was a useless farm dog, but Norman, who was a benevolent man, wasn't worried. Pip was a companionable dog and Norman forgave him his inadequacies.

If Pip had been a human, he would have been just the type of person that Norman avoided. Pip was always on the lookout to get something he shouldn't. He was sneaky, stealthy, and quite untrustworthy. You could see it in his eyes, which generally darted about seeking opportunities. He was always thinking. He was lean, as a lot of farm dogs were back then, and he tended to skulk and slink about, moving like he was made of liquid, curling himself quietly around doors and into places he shouldn't be, always alert, always looking for food.

Pip wasn't an extrovert like a lot of collies. He didn't jump up and smother you. He was not an in-your-face dog, not full of himself, but was generally friendly. He kept himself to himself and 99 per cent of the time he'd be fine. But there was always that one per cent there, meaning you just couldn't trust him completely.

Norman didn't expect too much of Pip, and Pip was an opportunist who would take any chance to grab food from whoever he could. Sometimes he was successful, managing to grab an egg here, a tart cooling on the rack there, or a farm worker's lunch which had been left carelessly unattended. Periodically, as a youngster, I'd hear the call. 'Pip! Get away with you!' And sometimes I'd see Pip streak past the house, a sandwich clenched in his jaws, often followed by

Early animals

a flying boot or a piece of farm equipment hurled hopelessly in his direction by a farm worker who anticipated a hungry afternoon without his lunch.

But these small and occasional hauls were nothing compared with Pip's finest hour, an audacious heist which went down in Manor Farm folklore as 'The day Pip got one over on Norman'. Although it is up for dispute, my grandfather may have had something to do with it, providing as he did an unwitting diversion behind which Pip carried out his dastardly act.

Norman and Fred were friends. Although Norman was technically Granddad Wright's boss, they got on well and would often stop each other for a natter, putting the world to rights or complaining about something or other – with Norman it would usually be the increasing price of cigarettes. On the day in question, a Sunday, Fred had walked past the farmhouse around midday on the way to check a calf that was under the weather and Norman was outside, having a cigarette in the garden because he didn't like to smoke in the house. Naturally, the men bid each other good day and started to chat.

'Morning Fred.'

'Morning Norman. I just called in to check on a calf I was worried about this morning.'

Norman explained that Joan had gone to church and that he'd managed to skip the Sunday service because he had urgent farm business to attend to, which was most likely reading the Sunday paper and enjoying a leisurely breakfast and a few Woodbines (cigarettes).

Fred noticed some mouth-watering aromas wafting through the open kitchen window. His stomach gurgled.

'Is dinner about ready, Norman? What are you having?'

'Well, Fred, I'm chief cook and bottlewasher while Joan has gone to chapel. We've got a lovely rib of beef. It's just resting on the side now. Puddings are in. I've got it all under control.'

It was then that Fred was momentarily distracted by a flash of black and white in the corner of his eye. He tilted his head to look past Norman, who was waxing lyrically about his prowess in the kitchen, to see Pip sprint away from the open back door, which led to the kitchen. Clenched firmly in the dog's jaws was a glistening joint of beef, still steaming, dripping with juices which had created a rivulet of reddish brown down his white chest – in fact, he looked like he was wearing a tie and bib. Pip's eyes were wide with excitement, basking in the ecstatic knowledge that he was making off with perhaps the biggest prize of his food-stealing career. Norman was in mid-flow of conversation and oblivious to his disappearing dinner. Fred, head still cocked to one side, narrowed his eyes and cleared his throat as Pip headed for the safety of nearby fields at one hundred miles an hour.

Norman stopped talking.

In classic Yorkshire understatement, Fred said: 'I think Pip's just had your dinner, Norman,' and pointed to the dog, who was now halfway across the field and moving at such speed that any attempt to catch him would be a pointless endeavour. Norman looked to where Fred was pointing and realised what had happened.

'The blessed dog!' he exclaimed, using the most restrained Methodist expletive he could muster. He ran off after the thief.

Granddad was still laughing about it several hours later when we all sat down to dinner in his cottage. We later heard that the verbal admonishments that were directed at Pip when he finally slunk back home later that afternoon with a full belly were nothing compared with the interrogation by Joan that Norman was subjected to for leaving the back door open while knowing what a thief Pip was.

Early animals

Granddad had a wonderful, dry sense of humour and loved a good laugh. He had the Yorkshire trait of being able to remain deadpan while he made a joke. Sometimes, he was so straight-faced while he was ribbing someone that they took him seriously, as was the case with one of the other characters in the village, Annie Hudson. She would often call in to my granny and granddad to ask for advice about something or other. She called Granddad 'master'. She came round one day when Granddad was sitting reading the paper.

'I've got a problem,' she said to Granny. 'I've got a hole in me nightie like that,' she explained, indicating the size of the hole by making a circle with her thumb and forefinger.

Granny told her not to worry as she had some spare material the same colour. She went into her sewing box and retrieved a sizeable patch of it.

Annie looked at it and exclaimed: 'Thank you, but it's a big piece of material for a little hole.'

Granddad put his paper down and, straight-faced, said: 'That's easy, Annie, all you have to do is cut the hole to fit the patch.'

Annie went away and did exactly as he said, not realising he was joking.

Anyway, back to Pip, who was one of the creatures in the village that I grew up in, as characterful as any of the human inhabitants. The story of the meat swoop is still recounted mirthfully today, even though Fred and Norman are long gone. While Pip wasn't a nasty dog by any measure, he could be unpredictable, and one day, when I was around seven and riding in the back of one of the farm vans with him, returning with Norman from a visit to the village shop for yet another packet of cigarettes, I reached over to stroke him. Quick as a flash Pip snapped out at me and caught my cheek with his teeth, drawing blood. I burst into tears, half from pain, half from shock. Pip wasn't a vicious dog but from then on, I learned to expect the unexpected from him and I also developed a healthy caution around farm dogs which has stayed with me to this day. With the benefit of hindsight, I realise that Pip would have been tired, hungry and probably a little anxious in the back of the noisy van, which he travelled in rarely, and, like anyone else in that situation, he lashed out because he wasn't in the mood for petting, being nonchalant about being stroked or fussed at the best of times. I'd picked the wrong moment and failed to read his mood. In the years since, I've become much more intuitive about animals and the moods they are in.

Border collies are highly intelligent, need a lot of exercise and if their requirements are not fulfilled, they can be quite erratic in their behaviour because they easily get bored. I'll frequently be at a farm on a job, bent over on the back of the car rummaging in the boot for equipment and something snaps on the back of my heels. I turn round and inevitably, there is a black-and-white dog that's had a nip at me and is running off. Collies are programmed to chase and to nip at heels, and sometimes don't care what they chase or what danger they put themselves in, particularly if they are bored and are looking for a job to do. On one farm I used to visit, there was a collie who couldn't distinguish between vehicles and livestock, or if he could, he didn't care and assumed it was his job to try and round up anything that was moving. When I left the farm, I'd look in my wing mirrors and see the lunatic hurtling down the access lane alongside me, feverishly barking, snapping at the wheels to herd me into one of the fields. On several occasions, when I slowed to avoid running him over, he'd manage to get his jaws on a hubcap and prise it off. When he was distracted, I'd drive off, making a mental note to pick up the hubcap on the next visit.

Early animals

He'd be there in the rear-view mirror, with a big silver disc in his mouth, looking confused. How he never broke his teeth was, to me, one of life's mysteries.

I can't recall a time in my life when there weren't animals around. In this beautiful part of the world which I am lucky enough to have been born and raised in, animals are part of the fabric of everyday life. My first memories are the sights, smells and noises of the animals on the farm and of the two- and four-legged feathered and furry friends that lived among us. As a toddler I remember wandering into the deep litter houses in my grandfather's garden where the family kept hens and chickens for meat. We sold the eggs to the locals and also supplied the local butcher with poultry. I loved watching them scratch and peck around and, as we lived next door to my grandparents, the sound of their clucking formed the soundtrack of my childhood. I never got too attached to any individuals because eventually they would disappear; it was just a fact of life that farm animals were food. There was no great issue about it. Farm folk are pragmatic, and although they were and are a caring, compassionate breed, they are not overly sentimental.

There were only around twenty houses in the village I grew up in dotted on either side of the single-track road which ran through it and finished in a dead-end. Vehicles were few and far between and so people were happy to let their animals roam free. Obviously, not everyone in the village was a farmer, but most had either pets or livestock, be they dogs, cats, chickens or even ferrets. One of our neighbours, Albert, owned a pack of seven dogs of all different breeds and varieties, which would wander up and down the road, cocking their legs against walls, gates and lampposts as they went. Albert was a retired builder from West Yorkshire, and he had a big rusty old van that he took his dog out in. When they knew they were going out, they became excited and bayed uncontrollably. The van probably should have been sent to the breakers yard many years before it finally gave up the ghost, but Albert kept it going with his rudimentary knowledge of mechanics and a degree of luck. It was held together with tape and the engine rattled and chugged and belched out black smoke. As he passed all you could hear was the cacophony of barking from the canine passengers scrambling around in the back. It must have been deafening for anyone unfortunate enough to be in the van with the dogs. Albert would wave through the steamed windscreen as he went. Eagle-eyed observers would notice that instead of the required tax disc in the windscreen, Albert had taken a pop bottle label with a similar design to the official disc and carefully cut it into a circle, and this was placed inside the tax disc holder.

Country pursuits were a big part of village life and that meant some practices that today certain people would find distasteful, particularly city folk who may not be as acquainted with rural ways from days gone by. These pursuits included rabbiting with ferrets. It was common for men – it was mainly the gentlemen – to keep ferrets, which would be sent down rabbit holes to scare the rabbits out. They were then caught and either sold to the local butcher or cooked at home. While some folk might recoil in horror at the thought of eating a cute floppy-eared rabbit, it was actually very common until a few decades ago. You could buy fresh rabbit in Sainsbury's, and it is still a dish that you find on some menus. In addition to providing locals with a tasty treat for the weekday casserole pot, rabbiting was also an effective and efficient method of pest control, which helped farmers protect their crops and kept the ferrets in a job.

Rabbiting was often done in pairs and provided the men of the village with an outdoor social activity long before golf became

Early animals

the go-to male weekend pastime. They would simply find a rabbit warren, peg nets over the boltholes and then send the ferrets in. The fleeing rabbits caught in the trap would be swiftly dispatched with a knock over the head and then either taken home for dinner or sold.

There was a time when lots of people living in the countryside would keep ferrets and go rabbiting, my dad being no exception. He kept them in a hutch in an outbuilding and they weren't considered pets as such, they were working animals. They didn't need to be trained. They were quick, agile and intelligent and would get excited when they were taken out in their wooden carry boxes because they knew what was about to happen.

One of my dad's occasional rabbiting partners was the village egg man, George Barker, who kept hens. Mr Barker did not smile much and was renowned for being thrifty. If Mr Barker could get one over on a customer by packing one less egg than ordered, he would. He was the type of person who gave even parsimonious Yorkshiremen a bad name. Hence, when Mr Barker went rabbiting with Dad, he was in it for the money, pure and simple, not the sport, the conversation, or the camaraderie. When those rabbits darted out of their holes, Mr Barker saw pound signs caught in the nets. For him, the sound of a rabbit being struck on the head was the sound of the till ringing.

On one of their outings, Mr Barker was particularly keen to bag himself several rabbits, which he had already planned to sell to the butcher in the town, who regularly took game to sell from the hunting fraternity. On this particular expedition it was left to my dad to put the nets securely over the boltholes. Mr Barker had already identified a network of burrows in pastureland and had asked the farmer for permission to rabbit there. The farmer was only too pleased to have someone deal with the increasing rabbit population. Mr Barker and my father trudged off with Mr Barker's ferrets and nets, and when they reached the hunting ground, Dad quietly went from hole to hole, carefully placing nets over each one. The nets are supposed to be held in place by pegs, and some people will also establish a second line of entrapment by encircling the whole warren with a ring net.

With the nets in place, Mr Barker opened the carry box in the middle of two holes which had not had nets placed over them. His two ferrets poked their heads out, sniffed the air and then scarpered underground, one in one hole, one in the other. Mr Barker stood back from the boltholes out of sight with a lead truncheon in his hand, ready to strike.

He called to my dad.

'Stand back, Ken, so you don't disturb them when they bolt. We don't want to lose any.'

For a few seconds all the men could hear were the scratching noises underfoot as the ferrets twisted through the network of tunnels. Suddenly there was squeaking which got louder until a ball of grey fur shot out of one of the holes with a net over it. But rather than get tangled up, it ran under the net and out into open grassland where it made a dash to a hedgerow, into which it disappeared. Seconds later there was another chorus of high-pitched squeaks and another escapee from another hole which zoomed effortlessly under another net. My dad realised he'd not pegged the nets down properly and scrambled to try and rectify the mistake just as another rabbit appeared and got away. It was too late then. The burrow was clear. Rabbits 3, ferrets 0. Dad could see the funny side and started laughing. Mr Barker on the other hand was bereft. As my dad told me later, poor old George had tears in his eyes.

Early animals

'He says, "You lost me two Bob there, Ken,"' Dad said as he laughed. 'I thought he was going to cry or burst a blood vessel.'

In Dad's opinion it was just desserts for the times when Mr Barker had tried to get one over on us. Only a few weeks previously when I was sent to him for a dozen eggs, he sent me home with eleven, and when I was told by Mum to mention the miscount the following week, he explained: 'No. Tell your mother I remember those eggs, and one on 'em wor a double-yolker.'

As I got older and started to explore the village and the surroundings on my own, I took regular trips to Manor Farm, where my favourite animals were the cows. There was something very peaceful and comforting about them. People misunderstand cows and think they're boring and stupid but when you look in a cow's eyes you can tell they are thoughtful creatures. I learned at a very young age that different cows on the farm had different personalities and characteristics. Some were sociable and trotted over to see me when they started to learn I always had a handful of feed, others were wary and more nervous. I used to love going to see the cows and letting them take food out of my hand. Those early interactions are what started my lifelong love of farming and working with farm animals.

My first real pet was a rabbit called Spot who used to get let out of his cage and would go tottering around the village, sniffing around and then would come back when he'd had enough. He was quite capable of finding his way home and as there was rarely traffic on the road through the village, he was quite safe. Indeed, his untimely demise was nothing to do with cars. Sadly, he met his end when he wandered into a field with some bullocks in it and got trampled.

I learned about the animals around me; I learned how to look after them and what they ate; I learned about their personalities and habits; and I learned to respect them. In those days people didn't dote on their animals in the way they do today but they were still compassionate and caring. No one wanted to see an animal suffer.

The other animal characters that all farms had were farm cats, vital for keeping the rodent population in check. Some lived in outbuildings, while others were lucky enough to be invited in and live indoors. We had several at home over the years. They'd get milk from the dairy cows and supplement their diets with the mice and rats they caught. They were never bought and sold, they just turned up at farms or had always been there. Our cats were brilliant opportunists who realised that their lot was improved if they proved themselves useful to humans, in much the same way as wild cats were domesticated many thousands of years ago. They were drawn to grain storages by the resident mice when humans became settlers and farmers, and then were encouraged to stay because they served a purpose.

Unfortunately, the farm cats of my youth had a lot of problems because they were territorial, and feline families stayed on the same farms and interbred. There was also a lot of feline flu that they passed on from one to the other, so they had chronic snuffles.

Feline leukaemia, which couldn't be tested for back then, was also a constant problem with farm cats. It could manifest as solid cancerous masses, and we lost one or two of the cats we had at home at a young age to this condition. I recall we had one kitten we took in with cerebellar hypoplasia, a neurological disorder that affects balance and coordination. The little mite would take a few steps and its back end would just painlessly flop over. It would then pick itself up and off it went again. It looked comical and just meant the cat appeared very clumsy and somewhat drunk.

I had an idyllic upbringing. People had a lot more time for each other and our tiny village was a real neighbourhood. People were

Early animals

multi-skilled; they kept hens for eggs, pigs for meat, goats for milk. They sold eggs and rabbits like George Barker did, or they took on odd jobs; for instance, my granddad would cut the local men's hair with a set of old hair clippers he kept in a metal Oxo tin. He wasn't trained; he taught himself. Hairstyling for men at that time was fortunately neither requested nor provided around the village.

The animals in the village were an integral part of my way of life, and through the people around me and my parents I learned how to look after them. I began to understand that occasionally, an animal would become ill or need something that the villagers could not provide, and in that case, a man turned up in a brown coat and a big pair of Wellingtons (large rubber boots) to fix the problem (inevitably back then it was a man, not a woman). That man was the vet, and when the vet came there would often be much sucking of teeth and knitting of brows because when the vet came out, it meant a bill would follow. Some farmers would make it their life's work to try and reduce their veterinary bills to next to nothing. Vets were respected, but also slightly begrudged because they came at a price. There was plenty of banter between farmers and vets, and an awareness of an uneasy symbiosis that neither could survive without the other. Little was I to know in those tender early years when I watched wide-eyed as the man in the brown coat administered to my bovine friends as they were calving, that one day it would be my arm inside the back end of a cow.

2

Wet behind the ears

Slowly and carefully, I ran the scalpel down the dog's shaved sternum. The flesh yielded to the knife and parted slightly to reveal the subcutaneous fatty tissues and the muscles and bone underneath. There was no blood. The dog was long since dead.

I was at Liverpool University School of Veterinary Science and was concentrating on dissecting a canine cadaver in one of the anatomy classes. The room was equipped with around twenty operating tables. On each was a dog, on its back. Around each table stood two students who were taking turns to examine their specimens. The room was quiet except for the occasional hushed whisper as the students concentrated on their tasks.

Just as I reached forward for a bone saw to open the ribs, something cold, sticky and wet hit the back of my neck.

Flup!

It stuck there for a moment, like one of those sticky children's toys that cling to windows when you throw them and then slowly climb down the surface as they begin to unstick. I was startled for a second and automatically reached round to pluck whatever it was away from my skin. When I looked at the orb of tissue it was easy to surmise what it was. One of the poor specimens had been deprived of a testicle, which had then been launched in my direction. As I examined it between thumb and forefinger, everyone else in the room had their heads down, including the culprit, so it was impossible to tell where it had come from.

Professor King, who was taking the class, sighed. He'd noticed what had happened and had seen it all before.

'Settle down please students. The anatomy of the testicle isn't until next week,' he said wearily.

At vet school, students didn't attend to a sick animal until the fourth year of the course. The dog dissection was one of the practical lessons in the first-year comparative anatomy module. The limited supply of specimens for the classes were stray dogs that couldn't be found homes. Sadly, there were packs of stray feral dogs roaming the streets of Liverpool city centre which were rounded up and euthanased. It was not unusual at that time for strays to end up at places like vet schools where they were used for science and study.

As the supply of animals was limited, the dogs had to be used for several dissections, concentrating on a specific part of the body each time. After each practical, be it a shoulder dissection, an eye or a chest, each specimen was placed back in the chiller and kept cold for another day. After about five or six days dissecting the same dog, however, they started to turn a bit ripe. Sometimes body parts would disappear and reappear later in the day on someone's plate in the refectory in the halls of residence, where I lived in the first year of my studies.

The humour was morbid at times but was good-natured and helped cope with the pressure of exams and coursework, which included subjects such as animal husbandry, animal welfare legislation and nutrition, which was studied on a biochemical level. I can still remember the Krebs citric acid cycle, which describes what happens in the liver when certain foods are broken down to release energy.

My favourite subject was parasitology, the study of parasites, which I was fascinated by. Our lecturer was a chap who taught at the nearby School of Tropical Medicine, which was in Liverpool because the city was a major seaport. In days gone by, ships would come in to the port from far-flung corners of the Earth, carrying exotic cargo. Along with the goods and commodities from far-off lands, the ships also brought in crews, and sometimes they carried diseases.

Parasitology was taught by a chap called Professor Beasley, and he was fanatical about the subject. He spoke passionately about different worms and their life cycles, how they latch onto gut walls with their teeth and reproduce. He was quite sentimental about some of the species he described.

'This lovely little job is the tapeworm *Taenia multiceps*,' he told us, smiling as he put a slide on the projector.

He looked like an archetypal academic with a big shiny bald dome, wisps of hair above his ears and a long nose. We disrespectfully called him Beaky Beasley but he was just the sort of bloke you wanted teaching you because he was enthusiastic.

He had a knack of bringing any conversation back round to parasites. If he was talking about his holidays, he would start to talk about the parasites he'd seen on his travels. His enthusiasm rubbed off on me and I became fascinated with parasites too. I'd be hard pushed to choose a favourite; it's like asking someone to choose their favourite child. I do have a soft spot for tapeworms, though.

Taenia multiceps is a lovely little tapeworm that lives in the small intestines of dogs. Its eggs are released in the dog's faeces which fall onto the ground. Grazing animals such as sheep ingest the eggs and become the intermediate host. The eggs hatch into larvae that migrate to the brain, eye or any other nervous tissue, causing cysts and a condition called circling disease, colloquially called Gid. The cysts continue to enlarge in the brain causing softening of the overlying skull. Affected sheep become disoriented and can often be seen wandering around fields in circles. In days gone by, farmers would sometimes perform their own curative procedures on these animals using an implement that looked like a bicycle pump with a spike on the end. The point would be used to penetrate the softened part of the skull and the liquid containing the larvae would be sucked out of the cyst. Some were cured. Most died. It used to be quite common in Wales, but the practice has thankfully died out now, as has the disease, mainly because dogs are now regularly wormed.

Even as a student I had pets, namely Ratty the rat, who was given to me by one of my fellow students and who used to sleep in a cage in the house I lived in when I moved out of the hall of residence. Ratty was a real character and used to enjoy Ribena and shortbread. I had Ratty for two years and missed him when he passed away very suddenly. His cage was on a table by my bed and one night, seconds after I switched off the light for bed, I heard a thump and thought he'd knocked something over. When I leaned over and switched the light back on, he was lying on the floor of his cage, legs in the air, completely motionless. I may not have been qualified at that stage, but I knew he was dead. Poor old Ratty must have had a heart attack and had died instantly. I buried him in the garden of the house, which backed on to Toxteth Cemetery, so at least he was in good company.

Even before I was a student, I often did work experience at Donald Sinclair and Alf Wight's veterinary practice at 23 Kirkgate in Thirsk, made famous in the books that Alf wrote under the pen name James Herriot. In the books, Kirkgate formed the basis of the fictional practice, Skeldale House, made famous in the TV series *All Creatures Great and Small*.

Donald, Alf, and Alf's son Jim, who later became my business partner in the real-life Skeldale practice that featured in *The Yorkshire Vet*, were all encouraging and allowed me to gain valuable hands-on experience with their patients. I would often go out on routine jobs with them, or one of the other vets who worked at Kirkgate, and, if they were lambing, they'd turn to me and say: 'Have a feel in here, Pete, see what you think.'

I'd tentatively insert a hand, and then an arm, and feel around inside the uterus, searching for legs and a head, and trying to work out which position the lambs were in and how many there were. The experience was invaluable.

One of the common procedures I was allowed to practise was pregnancy diagnosis, or PD, which could accurately be done manually from when a cow was as early as six weeks in calf. The vet feels for different things depending on the stage of pregnancy, and in order for the farmer to better manage his herd, the earlier the farmer knows a particular cow is in calf, the better. I learned that early PDs involve the vet inserting their hand in the cow's rectum and feeling the uterus through the rectal wall. Alf and Jim allowed me to perform this technique when I was a student.

Whenever they were called to do a PD (in those days it was sometimes only for two or three cows, whereas now my record is ninety-seven in one day) the farmer would stand by like an expectant father, always ready with an opinion. Early PDs could never be 100 per cent accurate, and vets would sometimes get it wrong. When they did, farmers delighted in reminding them of their errors. Like a lot of things in life, PDs were about practice. The more you did, the better your PD skills became, and I was given a very good grounding before I qualified from university thanks to the opportunities Alf and Jim gave me during my periods of work experience.

While most of the calls I accompanied the vets on were routine, some were out of the ordinary and stuck in my memory. The memory of one house call to attend to a dog at an old people's bungalow still makes me shudder.

We went to the address and knocked on the door. There was no reply, but I could hear the dog weakly barking inside. The door was open, so Jim pushed it and tentatively went in. The putrid smell that was already evident outside made us both hesitant.

'Hello? Are you there?' Jim called.

We took a few steps further into the hallway. I looked around, taken aback by the squalor of the place. There was rubbish everywhere and the stench became stronger. The carpet was sticky underfoot. Everywhere I looked there were old dirty bits of clothing, household waste, discarded packaging and rotting food, all left to gather dust or decay. The house looked like it hadn't been cleaned in years. Every surface was covered in dust, and it hung in the air. There was no colour in the house. Everything appeared to be a dull hue, as if any life and vibrancy that had once been in the space had been washed out. It was oppressive.

When we heard a frail voice coming from the sitting room, I didn't know whether to be relieved that the occupant was alive or horrified that someone was living in such awful conditions. We looked at each other, and although neither of us said anything, we both knew what the other was thinking. It was grim.

Inside the living room there were various pieces of furniture straining under the weight of piles of old magazines, books, newspapers, clothes, old bedding and towels. A sagging mattress was placed over two old chairs which were piled with blankets and sheets. At one end of this makeshift bed a woman's head appeared from under the covers. She had a beard of long grey whiskers and grey straggly hair. She looked pale, a gaunt apparition.

'She's over there,' she said, beckoning to the other side of the room with a bony finger.

There was another chair under a grimy window onto which had been heaped a pile of dirty old coats. A wretched-looking collie cross lay on top of them. Pus was dripping from her rear end and pooling on the floor. She was suffering from pyometra, an infection of the uterus. It was evident from the poor animal's condition that she was in the advanced stages. The dog was close to death and the old woman looked like she was too.

'We need to take her back to the surgery,' Jim explained, 'but we're probably going to have to put her to sleep because I don't think she's going to be strong enough to survive an operation.'

The lady nodded sadly. She understood how ill her companion was.

As we were carrying the poor dog away, I turned to Jim.

'We can't leave her like that,' I said.

'You're right there, Pete, we can't,' he agreed. 'I'll have a word with social services.'

The poor dog was beyond help and did have to be euthanased. Jim's sister was a GP and he told her about the old woman, and she reported the matter to social services who went round to help her.

Later, Jim took me aside.

'That wasn't a pleasant experience, Pete,' he said, 'but as a vet, you never can be sure what you'll stumble upon, and you have to be ready for anything.'

Wet behind the ears

By the time I graduated I had as much hands-on (or hands-in) experience as any other student on my course in Liverpool thanks to my work experience at 23 Kirkgate. The majority of students planned to go into a mixed practice dealing with all kinds of animals after graduation. In those days that was a normal career path as there wasn't a great deal of specialisation. Mixed practices dealt with small and large animals to a lesser or greater degree and were the backbone of the profession. The rural practices with farm clientele treated more large animals, while the urban and suburban practices dealt with more small animals. The majority of specialised practices were equine veterinary practices, and if a dog or cat needed specialist treatment it was often referred to a university.

After graduation, I approached the job market with trepidation as for some reason I've always felt inferior and have a deep-seated fear of failure; I think that comes with having a glass-half-empty outlook on life. I've always been a pessimist, but I can also see the positives of having a dour outlook, as the fear of failure has always driven me on.

In the event, finding work was not a problem. One of my friends from Liverpool was working at a practice in Harlow, in Essex. They were looking for someone on a short-term basis and I went to work there for a couple of months. After that I got a permanent job in a mixed practice called Kemble and Pinney in Luton, Bedfordshire, which was a big, busy practice with two branches serving a mixture of clients: farm, equine and small animals. The salary was £5,000 a year and the position came with a Ford Fiesta company car and accommodation above the surgery.

It was the early eighties, and the partners were forward-looking, having invested in the latest equipment and training. They did their own pathological tissue analysis whereby a human pathologist came in once a week to look at samples. They also had a laboratory with blood analysers at a time when most practices sent their samples to an external laboratory.

I still remember the first operation I carried out as a newly graduated vet. It was a cat spay, and just my luck, the patient was a stroppy one. Nowadays the anaesthetic is often given intramuscularly, which is easy because you can do it quickly and don't have to fiddle around. But back then the anaesthetic was administered intravenously into the cephalic vein that runs down the cat's forelimb. This meant you had to locate the vein and restrain the patient while you fiddled around with the needle. At that stage of my career, I was ham-fisted, and the nurse did her best to hold the cat as I tried to find the vein, which is only around three or four millimetres in diameter, while the cat became increasingly agitated and uncooperative.

After a minute of fumbling, the cat was in no mood to allow me anywhere near her, vocally making her disgust with me quite clear. My boss at the practice, Owen Pinney, was in the operating theatre next door, and although I was loath to disturb him and admit defeat, I knew I had no choice because this cat was never going to cooperate for me.

I went sheepishly into Owen's operating theatre. He looked up from one of the many intricate surgeries that he regularly carried out.

'Um. . . I'm sorry to bother you, but I'm having a bit of trouble giving an intravenous GA induction to a cat; she's getting a bit upset with me,' I offered as a gross understatement. 'Would you be able to bail me out, please?' I asked.

'Is it a black-and-white one?' Owen inquired.

'Yes. Why?' I replied. 'Do you know her?'

'No, but they're nearly always the stroppy ones,' he told me, laughing.

Owen came in and administered the anaesthetic within seconds and the bad-tempered cat drifted peacefully to sleep. The rest of the operation was uneventful, and the patient made a full recovery, but from that day on I did realise that Owen was right. For some unknown reason it is generally the black-and-white cats that have a tendency towards ill-temper.

I stayed at Kemble and Pinney for a year and it provided me with an excellent grounding for my future career and a wealth of experience with all species of animals. It was immensely busy and set me in good stead for my future career in North Yorkshire.

Kemble and Pinney was so busy that there wasn't much time for anything other than work. I was rushed off my feet every working day and noticed that within a few months of starting, despite being lean at that time, I had lost over half a stone in weight.

I lived in a very basic flat above the branch practice in Dunstable, which seemed a million miles away from the rural ideal of North Yorkshire. This living arrangement made it easier when I was on call during the night. Initially it was quite a lonely experience but then I was introduced to Morris. He was a stray cat that turned up at the surgery one day. Someone found him, didn't know what to do with him, and brought him in, which was a normal occurrence and still is when people find strays. Normally they would be sent to the local cat home or the RSPCA, or often one of the vet nurses would take them. But Morris looked at me, and I looked at him, and I couldn't resist the adorable little glint he had in his eye. He was only a kitten, an ordinary domestic shorthair, but I could tell he was imploring me to take him with me.

'Come on then,' I said as I laughed.

Initially I planned to keep Morris for a couple of weeks in case he had an owner who might show up to claim him. No one did and I was in no hurry to send him off for rehoming. Morris was in no hurry to leave either. He loved being in the flat and he loved me. He was a tonic to have around. He was always happy and playful. When I used to go back to my flat above the surgery after a day at work, I would hear the pitter-patter of his paws as he ran across the wood floor to meet me. No matter what kind of day I'd had, it was a brilliant sound to hear and always made me smile. As I was living on my own he was always so welcoming regardless of the mood in which I came home. He was my mate and we understood each other perfectly.

I don't understand people who say cats don't have personalities. Only someone who's never had a cat can claim they don't. They are expressive and they make their feelings perfectly clear. They get attached to their owners and become possessive of their households. For me at the time, Morris was the perfect pet. Like most cats, he pleased himself and was very independent, which was just as well as I wasn't around much to shower him with attention. He was quite happy on his own and the flat was his territory. Cats are solitary creatures generally and not inclined to share their quarters with too many others. I've often observed in multi-cat or cat-and-dog households that although it appears on the surface that everyone is living in harmony, when you look carefully, you'll see that the cats will all have their own territory that they stick to, where they are often much happier minding their own business.

I often find one will be living in the conservatory, one might live in one bedroom, while another lives in the sitting room. They often prefer not to have close contact with each other. They're quite happy to keep themselves to themselves and have you to themselves too. The times I've seen when they do share space comfortably and successfully are when there are two siblings or two that have grown up together from kittens. It's advisable to think carefully when planning to introduce another pet, be it a cat or dog, into a household where a cat is already established.

Morris lived with me all the time I was in Luton, and when I moved to Thirsk to work at 23 Kirkgate he came with me but sadly disappeared soon after the move. I never discovered what happened, whether he decided he didn't like the country life and scarpered or whether he was taken by a fox or befell some other misfortune. It was not knowing what happened to my good mate that was so painful.

Kemble and Pinney had several farm clients which I always enjoyed seeing, and I had many 'firsts' with them, including my first calving, which proved a far from simple challenge.

The farmer had called reception to request an urgent call-out, as one of his cows was struggling to give birth. Although I'd not calved a cow on my own before, I had assisted many with Alf and Jim and observed even more. I was slightly apprehensive to be doing it on my own, but I had also come across most of the eventualities I might be facing, so I took the job and drove my Ford Fiesta to a farm in rural Bedfordshire a few miles outside Dunstable with a degree of confidence but also a little nervousness.

The location was idyllic. A quiet canal ran through the pasture on which a small dairy herd grazed. The farmer met me as I pulled up in the yard and explained that he had tried to pull the calf out earlier but realised there was a problem and he wasn't sure whether the calf was dead or alive.

'I couldn't feel anything moving,' he said.

I was beginning to learn at that early stage of my career that one of the most important tricks a young vet could learn was the ability to appear supremely confident while masking a deep-seated sense of self-doubt.

I puffed up my chest slightly, looked him square in the eye and said: 'You did the right thing in ringing for my help.'

He nodded. I'd managed to fool him.

I then turned my attention to the patient and offered up a silent prayer. *Please let this be simple*, I thought.

Once my arm was inside and I could get a good feel around, I realised that the situation was anything but simple.

'It's all under control,' I reassured the farmer, who was standing passively nearby, arms crossed.

The calf was facing the right way with its legs forward, but its head was back, looking over its shoulder. There was no way it was coming out without help. I knew that if calves in these situations were small, it could be relatively easy to manoeuvre them into place, but I could tell this was a big calf. I reached as far as I could, with my arm almost up to my shoulder so I could run my hand along the arc of its neck. I was straining and breathing hard, but still trying not to let the farmer see just how how much I was struggling. Straining every sinew in my arm, I could just feel the nearest ear over the crest of the head. *Stay calm. Don't panic*, a little voice inside my head urged. I thought for a minute and pulled my hand back to the legs.

'Everything alright?' the farmer asked.

'Yes, I'm making progress,' I replied in as confident a manner as I could muster.

I held a foot and strained to pull the forelegs what seemed like millimetres, to try and bring the body and head forward towards me. Then I reached back along the chest and over its neck to the head. I was behind the cow with my arm so far inside her uterus that my head was bent to the side and my ear was pressed hard against her anus. Veterinary work can rarely be described as dignified!

The extra few millimetres I'd managed to gain helped because I could feel part of the way down the side of the calf's face and get to its eye. When I did, the calf blinked.

Not wanting to count my chickens, I exclaimed: 'It might just still be alive.'

'Well, I wasn't expecting that,' said the farmer. 'I thought we'd be lucky to save the cow.'

I then remembered something Alf Wight had said to me when we were at a similarly difficult calving.

'You can sometimes get your finger into the eye socket to pull the head round,' he said.

With his words of advice ringing in my ears, I stretched my index finger, found the outside edge of the eye socket where there is some room to get purchase, hooked my finger in and tugged. It would have been uncomfortable for the calf undoubtedly but there was no risk of damaging the eye. At this point I was panting with exertion with sweat pouring down my face.

'Do you need some help? I can always ring the practice and get one of the partners out,' the farmer asked. What an indignity! He knew I was young and obviously was not as confident in my abilities as I hoped he thought I was.

'No thank you,' I replied. 'I'm winning.'

Inside I was panicking.

'Come on, Peter, shake yourself, you can do this,' I told myself.

I pushed my hand in deeper, got a better grip in the eye socket, and pulled hard. I felt the head move slightly round. My heart leapt. Maybe this was going to work. Every tendon and sinew on my forearm sang and strained as I continued to pull. The head moved further. I carried on pulling for what seemed like an eternity, with me dripping sweat as, inch by inch, the head came round. When I was confident that I'd moved it enough, I released my hold and felt further along the face until I reached the calf's nose. The nostrils provided the next handhold.

Once again, I strained to pull the head the right way round.

'Is it still alive?' the farmer piped up. 'Are you sure you don't want me to call for some help?'

'If you'll just bear with me,' I said, as politely as I could.

It took several more agonising minutes but eventually, with a lot of tugging using muscles that had long been exhausted, I got the head facing forward towards me. By which time I was soaked in sweat. The relief was immense, and with everything in the right order I was able to get my rope around the back of the ears and through the mouth and pull the calf out. I lowered it onto straw, and rubbed it vigorously as it took its first breath. What a wonderful sight. In a split second I went from panic to elation.

The farmer looked on and managed a smile.

'I didn't think you were going to be able to do that,' he said.

'No, it was a bit tricky, but the outcome was never in doubt,' I lied.

I soon learned that no two days were the same and that you could never second-guess what would walk through the door or what you'd find on a farm visit.

At Kemble and Pinney I saw the worst case of parasites I've ever encountered. A dog was brought in because it could not stop vomiting and obviously had some form of blockage in its gut. It was a very young puppy, just a few weeks old. We couldn't work out what was causing the problem, and nothing showed up on an X-ray. Despite my best efforts the poor thing died, and we examined it to find out the cause of death. When we opened it up we found that it had so many roundworms in it that they had balled together in its intestine like a rubber-band ball, and this had caused the obstruction.

As a mixed veterinary practitioner we inevitably were asked to attend a variety of species, not just cats and dogs, and towards the end of my time in Luton I was asked to see an African Grey parrot that needed his nails clipped.

Its owner, an elderly lady, called the surgery and requested the last appointment of the day.

'It's a bit embarrassing,' she confessed. 'I'd rather bring him in when no one else is there because he uses a bit of bad language.'

I was on duty that day when she came in at the end of a long shift. To be honest I was quite looking forward to meeting this foul-mouthed bird after what had been a fairly mundane day. The lady placed him on the examination table and removed the blanket that was covering his cage.

'Hello,' I said. 'Who do we have here?'

I was secretly hoping for a stream of comical expletives, but the parrot just looked at me quizzically and blinked, unfazed.

Parrots have powerful beaks and have to be handled with great care. He was a big chap, so I asked one of the nurses to assist. She put on a big pair of gauntlets that we kept for handling risky patients and reached into the cage where she held the bird and pushed him carefully up against the side of the cage where I could get to his claws and clip them through the bars.

The parrot was not happy with this arrangement and squawked but still made no utterance.

I held the clippers with one hand, got hold of one of his toes with the other, and just as I was about to clip the first nail he let out his uncompromising comment.

'Get off yer bugger!' he screeched. I had to stop momentarily because I was laughing so much. The comic timing was perfect. The task was completed without a hitch and without my new feathered friend making any further utterance. As I drove home to tell Morris about it I was still chortling.

3

Thirsk for knowledge

I returned home to Thirsk in 1982 relatively shortly after qualifying, following my short stay working as a qualified vet in Luton. After my studies and the period I spent in Luton, I came to a world that seemed like a bygone age compared with what I'd experienced. The animals were the same, but the practices and people belonged to another era when the pace of life was much more gentle.

I have kept some of the original day books from 23 Kirkgate, in which the activities of the practice were logged, and occasionally I bring them out to leaf through them. They provide a nostalgic meander down memory lane and act as time capsules, giving a good indication of the pace of life as it was then.

Two puppies. Remove retained baby teeth, reads one entry. This would have been a quick and simple job involving a whiff of gas to sedate the puppies and while they were asleep, one of the vets would prise the teeth out. It would have been over in no time as deciduous, or milk teeth, have very small roots on them. The cost of the procedure was listed as £15.

Booster. Horse, reads another. That job would have been done by Madeleine, one of the vets working at the practice at the time. She was also a Liverpool graduate and had completed her training three years before me and was the provider of my university friend 'Ratty'. The job would have involved a nice ride out to one of the stables or farms outside town and a simple injection.

Cox, Hambleton. Visit, X-ray, horse. That would have been an equine job for Donald Sinclair, one of my old bosses and a colourful character. In the Herriot books, Siegfried Farnon was based on Donald. He was a horse expert and the equine fraternity from far and wide would call on his services. He enjoyed his status within the horse community, who were generally a notch or two higher up on the social ladder in many cases. At Kirkgate we had a mobile X-ray unit that fitted in the back of a car but the operation of it would require two vets: one to work the machine and one to hold the plates in place behind whatever was being imaged.

One that always makes me chuckle is: *Cat stung by bee, visit as soon as possible.* I can't imagine any vet today paying a house visit to a cat that's been stung by a bee, unless there has been some kind of extreme allergic reaction and the cat has collapsed. But when I returned to Thirsk these were the sort of visits we were making within the practice. *Visit dog. Heart attack.* Then later: *Dead on arrival.* Donald and Alf would have shied away from anything like that because that sort of job could be a bit more technical and one that many a senior partner would swerve.

The list goes on. *Visit calf, swollen navel.* This would have been an infected umbilicus and would have involved a quick shot of penicillin and a follow-up to check the infection had cleared. The next entry, *Visit calf. Lump on leg*, would have been another job for Donald as it involved a pleasant ride out to Ampleforth on the

Thirsk for knowledge

edge of the beautiful North York Moors national park and a quick examination. Donald and Alf enjoyed the uncomplicated jobs, as indeed we all did. If there was anything strenuous to attend to, such as a castration or a difficult calving, Donald's practice partner Alf would wave his hands around mysteriously like a wizard and, with a grin on his face and a spooky voice say, 'I'm looking into my crystal ball here and I foresee a young fit man going out to castrate some energetic, large bulls.' He made no bones about passing on the more physically demanding jobs to us youngsters as he reached retirement age, and who could blame him?

One of my favourite clients at the time was also in Ampleforth. Ampleforth College Farm was situated in the grounds of a beautiful Benedictine monastery and famous boys school. The farm was an integral part of the monastery and school where they kept a herd of dairy cows to provide milk and dairy products to both. Any excess that the herd of around 250 cows produced was sold to local businesses such as The Harbour Bar in Scarborough (owned by a former pupil), where it was used to make delicious ice cream, or was sold to the Milk Marketing Board. The cowman who looked after the herd, John Dawson, was the font of all knowledge when it came to dairy herds. He also had a great sense of humour and enjoyed gently winding people up, including me.

One day he told me that another farmer nearby had visited him looking for advice for an unusual problem.

John explained: 'He came down to see me and he said to me, "John, I need your advice. I've a calf that headbutts the milk bucket whenever I put it down to feed him with it. I think 'e's got some sort of deficiency."'

Calves were reared on reconstituted powdered milk twice daily until they were weaned at around eight weeks of age.

John started chuckling.

'You and I know that it's just a naughty calf, but I told him that it sounds to me like the calf has a vitamin deficiency that's making it feel disorientated each time it lowers its head. "I've heard of this before," I said to him, and I gave him a shot of multi-vitamins and told him that ought to sort it out.'

The farmer, who'd never heard of this strange affliction before (mainly because it was completely made up), went away thinking he'd been given a great pearl of wisdom and administered the vitamins without delay.

'He came back a week later and he couldn't contain himself,' John said, laughing. '"By 'eck, John," he says, "you've cured that calf of its mental deficiency. It hasn't butted the bucket over since I gave him that jab of multi-vitamins."'

Visits in those days inevitably involved a chat, a nice brew and, if you were very lucky, a slice of cake. Life was simpler then and although the days flashed past, it was a more sedate pace of life than life today. There would be around fifteen to twenty visits a day on the busiest days, so even if cake was only provided on a third of those, it was still easy to expand your waistline. Tea and a natter were the rule of thumb wherever you went. Everyone at the practice had their favourite jobs and clients, and many of the clients had their favourite vets.

Alf was universally popular, not because of his James Herriot books, the first of which was published in 1972, but because he was an exceptionally good vet and one of the nicest men you could possibly meet. His clients included Jeanie and Stephen Green – the Thirsk stalwarts made famous on *The Yorkshire Vet*. They had only been married for four years in 1982 when I started work at Kirkgate.

Thirsk for knowledge

Alf put versions of many of his patients in his books, including the famously indulged Pekinese, Tricki Woo, whose real name was Bambi. He belonged to Mrs Pumphrey, who in real life was Miss Marjorie Warner, an aristocrat who lived in Sowerby in a beautiful home called Thorpe House, which was a manor house with sprawling grounds. She was aristocratic in the true sense of the word, and had her own manservant. Alf was regularly called to deal with Bambi's 'flop bot', a rather quaint name coined by Miss Warner to describe a rather unpleasant condition. Dogs have small scent glands on either side of the anus and every time a dog defecates, a little bit of liquid is squeezed out of these sacs which gives each dog a distinct odour. This is so that when a dog is out sniffing around, he can recognise the scent of other dogs. It's like a canine calling card and lets all the dogs in an area know who's been where. Sometimes these little sacs do not empty as well as they should and become overfull, causing irritation. In order to try and clear the backlog, dogs will often scoot along the ground on their backsides. People often think this comical-looking behaviour is caused by worms causing anal irritation. Bambi was regularly afflicted, and when he was, Miss Warner would call the practice and request a visit from 'Uncle Herriot' who would have to administer to Bambi and sort his 'flop bot' out, which involved emptying the anal glands by pulling the tail up to bring the sacs towards the anus and then getting his fingers behind them and squeezing out the fluid. If that didn't work, the sacs could be emptied by putting fingers into the rectum to express the glands internally.

Alf practically became Bambi's personal physician; no one else would do. He was a very particular dog. It wasn't for the likes of him to have common dog food. And when Miss Warner went away, she would never put Bambi into kennels. Neither would she leave him with her manservant. The only person who could be trusted was Uncle Herriot, and so the picky Pekinese would come to 23 Kirkgate where he'd share the lovely walled garden behind the practice with Donald's and Alf's dogs. For the first few days Bambi would look at his dog food and turn his nose up. *I'm not eating that rubbish*, he'd say to himself. But he soon learned that the other dogs would immediately devour it if it was left unattended. And so by about day three Bambi realised that if he didn't move sharp, there'd be nothing for him and he'd be hungry. Miss Warner always used to ask Alf what trick he'd performed because when Bambi returned home his appetite was phenomenal and he'd eat anything.

Bambi was grateful for the personal care he was afforded. One Christmas Alf received a Fortnum and Mason hamper from Thorpe House and when he wrote to Miss Warner to thank her, she was most indignant.

'That wasn't from me,' she scolded. 'That was from Bambi!'

From then on, the hampers arrived every year, and every year Alf would send a letter to *Bambi Warner Esq.* thanking him very much for the present.

Tricki became so famous through the James Herriot books that there is even a Tricki Woo Suite at Skeldale House in Askrigg, where the original *All Creatures Great and Small* series was filmed.

There was much to laugh about in those days and Donald was a constant source of amusement. He loved to work in the higher echelons, the hierarchy of the area. He was very much a part of the local equine and hunting fraternity and was a dapper *bon vivant*. One day I was out with him in his car, and he asked me to get a cloth for him out of the glove compartment to wipe the windscreen.

When I opened it, a pile of moleskins fell out.

'What are these for?' I asked.

Thirsk for knowledge

'I'm collecting them up to have a moleskin waistcoat made,' he replied, matter-of-factly. It was just one of the eccentricities that Donald was renowned for but completely unaware of.

Donald liked to keep up to date with news in the profession through our journal, the *Veterinary Record*, which he read avidly and would often wave around if he found an article that interested him. One day he read out a headline loudly.

'Veterinary Practice. Profitable Business or an Expensive Hobby?' he said.

Donald had been thinking. This was always a concern to the rest of us. Alf Wight would usually shrink away when Donald began espousing one of his theories.

'Look boys, I've been working it out,' he explained. 'Unless we take 58.6p a minute, we'll go out of business.'

This was the type of thing he would say regularly, and then come out with a hairbrained scheme to increase profit.

'Just take it with a pinch of salt,' Alf would advise. 'You know what he's like.'

But this particular article, which highlighted the financial pitfalls of veterinary practice, had grabbed his attention and put the fear of God in him. He called a meeting for the following day, and in the meantime, each vet at the practice was asked to list their jobs per day, price them up, itemise the bill, and then see what they'd brought to the practice coffers, to make sure that, to coin his phrase, the business wasn't 'going to the wall'. Donald used to worry about these sorts of things all the time. He was a constant worrier.

And so the following day, a Tuesday, we met in the office at 4pm after afternoon surgery, each with our list. Jim had been operating all day, Tim had been castrating bulls and doing pregnancy diagnoses, I'd been doing horse work all day, and we were all knackered. By

4.15 there was no sign of Donald, so Jim asked our receptionist, Joan, who was in the office, if she knew where he was.

'He's gone home,' she said.

'Is he coming back?' Jim frowned.

'No. He won't be in until the morning,' she answered.

This was typical Donald. Despite his fearful misgivings the previous day that the practice was going bankrupt, he'd completely forgotten about this urgent meeting. In his absence, we all looked at our cases, itemised them, costed them, and realised that everyone was more than earning their keep. Then we looked in the logbook at Donald's contribution to the practice coffers that day. There was only one entry; it read: 'Mrs Sellers. Visit budgie. Dead on arrival. No charge.'

This was so typical of Donald's baffling inconsistencies, showing utmost kindness despite twenty-four hours earlier claiming that the practice could be going bankrupt.

One of my favourite Donald stories involved his attempt to revive a dead cat, which played out like something from a Monty Python sketch. It happened many years before I returned to Thirsk but was one of the legendary stories that was told to all new recruits. Although black humoured, it was passed down from veterinary assistant to veterinary assistant. Donald had wandered into the operating room one day where a cat had sadly died after being administered anaesthetic. One of the vets was trying to revive it. Donald sprang into action immediately. Sometimes farmers will try to revive new-born lambs by swinging them by the back legs to expel fluids from their airways, thereby enabling them to breathe. Donald thought this method might work on the cat, so he grabbed it by the hind legs, went out into the garden and started swinging it around wildly. Unfortunately, Donald's grip was not tight enough. The limp cat slipped out of his hand and sailed over the six-foot high garden wall into the yard of the British Legion next door, where one of the cooks was sitting on the kitchen step peeling potatoes. He was most perturbed when a dead black moggy plopped on the ground in front of him. The cat, which had long since passed, was oblivious to this unintended indignity.

We never knew what had caused the poor cat's demise. Ether was commonly used as an anaesthetic in those days, the outcome of which was wildly unpredictable, sometimes causing profuse salivation and death.

Chloroform was also used in the field to anaesthetise horses. It also had its challenges. It was administered via a canvas muzzle that fitted over the horse's mouth and nostrils and was held in place with a leather strap that went over the horse's head. There was a sponge inside the muzzle, which was zipped from the front. A quantity of chloroform liquid was poured onto the sponge, the muzzle was zipped up and the vet then waited for the horse to drop down. If you were lucky, this would be in the field you were working in. Sometimes the horse lost consciousness several fields away, having bolted in the initial excitement phase that the substance appeared to sometimes induce. I've no proof to back this theory up but it's my contention that in those days vets would have made excellent fell runners, on account of the miles they clocked up chasing anaesthetised horses across fields. It was an uncertain endeavour to say the least; you were never quite sure where they were going to drop or indeed if they were going to succumb. It certainly was far from an exact science. There was no magic formula and the amount of chloroform needed varied from animal to animal. They'd eventually keel over, providing you'd given them enough, but sometimes they just staggered about and came round again, in which case the vet would have the more difficult task of upping the dose and repeating the procedure, but now with an extremely wary and skittish patient who was aware of what was coming.

With cows, sedatives were occasionally used for a fractious or difficult patient. For a caesarean section, for instance, the aim was to give just enough to relax your patient but insufficient to cause them to go down, because performing a caesarean section on a recumbent cow was hard work. Calves weigh anywhere between fifty and eighty kilos, and if the mother was on the ground, that's a dead weight that needed to be lifted working against gravity. It was much more efficient to let gravity work for you, hence caesarean sections are better carried out on a standing cow. Once the cow was suitably sedated, local anaesthetic was injected into the flank or the spine to numb the nerves supplying the flank area where the incision was made. You would then cut into the flank and the uterus to deliver the calf. The farmer would often refer to this method as 'through the side door'.

In the comfort of the practice, things were much more controlled, and for dogs we used a type of barbiturate which was administered intravenously to induce a patient. Once he or she went off to sleep a gaseous anaesthetic was administered via a tube placed down the patient's trachea, and this had a blow-up cuff to create a seal between the tube and the trachea. This allowed the assisting vet or nurse to control the depth of anaesthesia by adjusting the concentration of the gas.

Although I had enjoyed working in Luton, it felt right that I was returning to Thirsk and the Kirkgate practice that had given me my early work experience. I was returning home. The culture was very different, but it was one I was intimately familiar with. I knew the people of Thirsk, I knew their mentality, I was one of them, they were my people. Being a vet in a small market town like Thirsk can be challenging because when everyone knows everyone, and everyone gossips, reputation is everything and there was in some ways greater pressure not to make mistakes. As the saying goes, no news travels like bad news. In Luton I was just the vet. That was obvious. Whereas in a small market town and a community like ours, you're integral to that community, especially one in which you were born. This can work in your favour if you build a good reputation, but it can be a curse if you blot your copybook in any way. There is certainly a loyalty to vets, and people will follow them from practice to practice. As I have said many times, it was always a fear of failure that spurred me on to do the very best I could for my patients and clients alike.

Even though the James Herriot books and the television series *All Creatures Great and Small* had placed Kirkgate on the map by the time I started working there, we didn't have people queuing down the street because of the practice's fame. But people did come from far afield from places like Scarborough, Bridlington, Leeds, York and Harrogate, because they had friends in Thirsk who recommended us. The practice did well through word of mouth because of the service that we gave.

My favourite time then was lambing season. And it still is now. It's springtime, a time of new beginnings, hope and new life. I'll never, ever tire of lambing season and of seeing newly born lambs gambolling across fresh green pastures. They look so full of joy, and to me they signify the promise of life ahead, which is ironic really because there's a saying in farming circles that sheep have one ambition in life, and that's to die!

This I found to be true because they do find quite novel ways of dying. Often, I'll treat a sheep for something simple and innocuous and leave thinking, *That'll be better tomorrow*, only to receive a message a few hours later from the farmer saying: 'That sheep you treated, it died last night.' (Farmers delight in delivering bad news.) And I'd be left pondering, *Why? Why did she die? There was no reason for that sheep to die.* And of course, the answer is simple. She died because she was a sheep.

I witnessed the most bizarre illustration of this propensity to unnecessary and avoidable mortality several years ago. A flock of sheep were in a field. There was nothing in the field except grass and a single tree with a low bifurcation of the branches, forming a V-shape around four feet from the ground – sheep head height. One of the flock stuck its head in the V and hung itself. Why? It was the only thing in the field that it could possibly find to hasten its demise. And that's typical of sheep.

In another recent case I was called out to dehorn a Swaledale ram. These are lovely-looking animals with horns that curl round behind their ears and over the sides of the face. They look magnificent but sometimes these horns can grow too close to the face and can actually grow into the side of it, causing wounds and skin ulceration – a perfect example of a bred-in design fault. This particular ram was beginning to suffer from such an issue, and so I went along to give its horns a trim. When I arrived, the farmer had brought him off the hillside and had him in a trailer ready for me.

Trimming horns is not technically a difficult job (I use a cheese wire to saw through them), but you do need to be careful because if you take the horns too low, they can bleed profusely, and you can't numb them very well with local anaesthetic like you can when you dehorn cattle because the nerve to the horn isn't particularly accessible. Consequently, you have to sedate your patient and administer painkillers so they're woozy and semi-conscious and don't feel the pain of the procedure.

My patient in this case was a young, fit animal so I gave it a sedative, which seemed to work well. I could see that one horn had already ulcerated the skin quite badly. Dehorning adult rams such as this can result in severe haemorrhage, but these horns didn't bleed one little bit and I got them sufficiently far back so that all the face was free of the ingrowing horn. It was a textbook job, and I drove away from the farm knowing everything had worked perfectly, giving myself a pat on the back as I looked over at the ram sitting up in the trailer.

I went to work the following morning and was greeted by one of the vet nurses.

'We had a message from the owner of that ram you dehorned yesterday,' she told me. 'It died hours later.'

I threw my hands up and groaned the familiar lament.

'Why? Why did he die?'

There was no need. He was fine when I left. We both looked at each other and shrugged. No words were needed. We both knew the answer. He was a sheep, and sheep have a habit of dying, even when you are convinced they won't, as I was in this case.

Indeed, sheep are funny things. Most people only know them as little white dots in the distance as you drive through the countryside. Fluffy clouds on green pasture. We don't make a point of thinking too much about what goes on inside their heads and subsequently we tend to assume not much does. But they are gentle, thoughtful creatures. When you look in their eyes, you can see the cogs turning. They have an inner life and people who work with sheep grow to love them. Some become pets, particularly the ones that end up being hand-reared. This often happens as a result of simple mathematics. You see, a ewe has two teats, so it can only feed two lambs at a time. Ewes mostly have one or two lambs, which works out fine, but they can have up to four. In some cases, a ewe with a single lamb can sometimes foster another, but spares without a teat are often hand-reared by being bottle fed and referred to as pet lambs. These sometimes manage to enchant their carers and get saved from the roasting tin.

I used to look after one such ram named Norman. His owner has a smallholding, and he had become a family pet through this process. He came to me with a suspected broken leg, but when I X-rayed him, I discovered he had a cruciate knee injury, similar to the type of injury footballers sometimes sustain. I put him on a course of injections, and he recovered fantastically well. Norman was treated like royalty by his family and was waited on hand and hoof.

Once you get hooked on keeping sheep it can be hard to stop. I know one couple, Keith and Hazel, who wanted a few sheep to keep on their smallholding. They bought three or four pet lambs to rear by bottle from a local farmer. They grew up, and as they matured Hazel realised they all had their own personalities and idiosyncrasies, and had over time been given names such as Fluffy, Curly and Bandy Legs. They had lambs and they grew up. Hazel still couldn't bear to part with any of them. By the time the couple retired forty years later, they had several hundred sheep of all breeds grazing in fields all around the Thirsk area. She was addicted to the love of sheep and couldn't bear to think of any of her extended family going off to slaughter.

The moral of this tale? Be careful what you wish for, and never underestimate the magnetism of animals and particularly in this case sheep.

4

Risky business

The phone trilled on Joan Snelling's desk. She was the formidable gatekeeper at 23 Kirkgate and later came to work with me at my Skeldale practice. Joan started work at Kirkgate when she was sixteen years old in 1959, and by the time I returned there in the early eighties, she had established herself as the matriarch of the practice family. The vets liked to think they were in charge, but it was Joan who really ran the place. She was an expert at dealing with difficult customers, chasing late payments, and keeping everyone in line. She also used to oversee anaesthetics and sterilised instruments.

As a newly qualified vet she kept a close eye on me, and on this particular day she obviously decided it was time for me to take a step up the professional and social ladder.

The caller was from the 'higher echelons' of society, shall we say. She had called because one of her prize mares was lame. She wanted Donald because he had a well-deserved reputation as one of the best equine experts in the country. He would be called upon for all manner of horse business. He would regularly be asked to examine stallions for soundness to make sure they were fit. He had his own Cleveland Bays which were superbly bred, one of which he gifted to Her Majesty the Queen. He was well respected in equine circles. He regularly went hunting himself and had his own pack of harrier hounds.

His veterinary expertise in the horse world and prowess at hunting ensured that as a member of our profession he lived the life of Reilly (added to the fact that he married a lady of significant wealth). Donald spoke the same language as equine enthusiasts, and in the horsey set he was invariably the first-choice vet. He would travel long distances to see clients. People in the horse world respected an equine vet more in those days if they owned and rode their own horses. Some might call it snobbery. I just accepted it was the way the world worked. I didn't ride, at least not very well. I'd tried once, was not competent enough and decided that I wouldn't attempt to get any better for fear of making a fool of myself.

When Joan explained diplomatically to the caller that Donald was indisposed (he was off to lunch somewhere), the lady was audibly upset.

'But this is urgent,' she said. 'When will he be back?'

'Not for several hours,' explained Joan. 'Can I send one of our other vets?'

The caller sighed.

'Well, I don't have any choice, do I?' she huffed.

I overheard the call. I didn't have any calls to make or appointments for a couple of hours so when Joan put the receiver down, I hesitantly offered to go.

I was duly dispatched to the nearby estate, which had stabling for around ten horses. And I was met by the owner, who looked me

Risky business

up and down when I got out of my car with an expression as if she had just noticed something distasteful on the sole of her shoe.

'Who are you?' she said.

'I'm new. I've just come back to work at Thirsk,' I replied.

'This is no good. They've sent a boy to do a man's job,' she snapped.

I tried to be polite and professional, ever wary of building a reputation with clients.

'I'm very sorry, but Mr Sinclair isn't available today, he's otherwise engaged. Would you like me to go away?'

'You're here now. You might as well have a look at her,' the woman conceded.

She took me into one of the stables where a beautiful bay mare was standing with one front fetlock bent slightly to keep the weight off her foot. I bent over and slowly ran my hand down her leg from the knee to the hoof. I could feel a strong pulse to her foot, and the hoof felt quite hot.

This could be an abscess, I thought. *This might not be as bad as it looks.* A cautious feeling of relief swept over me and my confidence began to rise.

A lame horse can be a puzzle. Sometimes you haven't a clue what the problem is, and back then there was no scanning equipment available in general practice like there is today. If the problem wasn't easily apparent, you had to carry out nerve blocks to numb the areas of the limb and all sorts of things to try and work out where the issue lay.

I picked up the foot and squeezed the hoof firmly. The horse pulled away and stepped back, which suggested that there may have been an abscess under the sole of the hoof.

I could sense the piercing eyes of the owner and the tension building in the stable as I took out my hoof knife. Then I picked the foot up again and started to pare down into the sole at the painful point I had noted under digital pressure. I took great care, knowing that the area was sensitive and it would be painful if I cut into an abscess.

The horse, noting the tenseness of her owner, suddenly jerked her foot away again. I held on and as I did, my knife slipped and cut across my other hand. I tried to maintain a dignified air as I looked down and saw my own blood dripping from the sizeable gash in my hand onto the foot I was still holding. It began to pool on the floor.

From where she was standing, it looked to the woman as if the blood was pouring from the hoof.

She shrieked.

'What the hell have you done! You've cut her!'

Still in pain, I stammered to tell her the injury was mine, but she was shouting at me, and I couldn't get the words out.

'You idiot! I knew I should have waited for Sinclair. Oh God, what have you done?'

Her temper was rising. She started throwing her hands around dramatically.

'Please. . .' I stuttered. 'It's not—'

But I couldn't be heard over her indignant protestations.

'My mare!' she screeched. 'If you've damaged her, you'll pay!'

I raised my voice to make myself heard.

'Madam, please listen to me for a minute!'

Momentarily she was stunned that anyone would have the audacity to speak firmly to her and she stopped in full flow.

I raised my bloody hand to show her.

'The horse is fine,' I said. 'Look. It's me that's bleeding.'

She looked at my hand as the penny dropped. She was silenced for a split second before the next compassionate volley.

'Thank God for that,' she said, totally unconcerned by my injury. 'I thought you'd damaged the horse.'

After hastily cleaning and bandaging my own wound, I returned to work on the mare's foot and very quickly pared into the abscess to release what to me was the lovely sight of pus and not my own blood trickling onto the ground in front of me.

By that stage the woman had warmed slightly but was still totally unconcerned about my injury. It was as if she had erased the gash in my hand completely from her memory. The horse made a complete recovery, but despite my success, Donald remained the first-choice vet for that particular client in the future. A mercy that I was forever grateful for.

Farm work, I learned over the following months and years, can be a risky business.

A big hazard has always been cattle, especially beef suckler cows, which are cows that are left in the herd to suckle their young and rear them. There are two types of cows. Dairy cows produce milk and their calves are taken off suckling their mothers at a few days old. Beef cows are left to suckle until they are weaned and start grazing. Dairy cows are used to being handled because they are milked every day. Suckler cows aren't handled much at all and are generally bigger, and some certainly know how to throw their weight about. They have less contact with people. They can kick faster than a blink of the eye and can be difficult to deal with, particularly the hot-headed continental breeds like Limousin and Charolais, which will run through you given the opportunity. Treating them or routine testing them for tuberculosis, which must be done every four years in our area, is a task which can be described in the veterinary world as a 'bit of a rodeo', particularly if the restraining and handling facilities are not robust. It's the sort of job that Alf would always send his younger, fitter recruits out to do.

One farm we went to had suckler cows which we could not recollect ever seeing or treating, nor could the farmer recall bringing them indoors. Somehow, they appeared to have slipped through the Defra net for routine TB testing. One fateful morning an official looking letter thudded onto the door mat in the farmhouse to say the herd had to be TB tested. This involves a veterinary surgeon getting up-close-and-personal to the animal to inject a small quantity of a substance called tuberculin into the skin in the neck region. When I arrived, the farmer had managed to coax them inside with food over a two-day period but they were utterly wild. As I peered through the metal grill of the window in the brick building they were in, all I could see was a frothing, wide-eyed mob of cows with a common agenda to kill anybody who set foot inside with them. As I surveyed this sea of angry snorting faces my cowardice or, as I prefer to call it, self-preservation, kicked in. They were literally feral cows, lethal, and there was no way we could test them for tuberculosis.

Under Defra rules, any cows that were not or could not be tested for tuberculosis had to go for slaughter and could not enter the human food chain. This is one of the very few times in my life where I admitted defeat before even starting a task.

When dealing with cattle, vets are reliant upon the farmer having a good stock handling system in place, ideally a gated collection area, with a gated race where you can isolate an animal into a cattle crush and hold it there while you work on it. Unfortunately, the standard of the system varies widely between farms. Going back in time, many holding systems were held together by string, which was copious on farms and often referred to as binder twine, used for tying up hay bales. It was found either hanging up on a nail or in a farmer's pocket ready for use.

One of the most important lessons I learned was to stand sideways on to a cow or young bull because they kick at groin level, and the last thing you want is a kick in the nether regions. For large animals they can be extremely quick and agile, so you don't get a chance to move out of the way. I've been caught more times than I care to remember, and it always happens when you're least expecting it. Often, it's the quiet ones who don't look like they will be a problem who catch you out. Recently, I was caught low down on my shin twice in the same place. My leg was swollen for weeks afterwards.

Kicks are not the main danger, however. In fact, bulls don't really kick. It is their heads and powerful necks you must be careful of. A full-grown male bull's head is the animal equivalent of a wrecking ball, topped with spikes if it has horns. The damage this bovine flail is capable of can be catastrophic. I know of several farmers who have been very badly gored and even killed by bulls and one colleague recently who has been permanently paralysed. Dairy breed bulls are known for being more aggressive than beef breeds such as Angus or Shorthorn, but I have learned to treat them all with great respect.

Breeding bulls, otherwise known as stock bulls, have got to be in tip-top condition and have got to have good feet, particularly the rear feet, as they've got to be able to stand on them comfortably when they are mating cows. For this reason, farmers always try to ensure that their stock bulls' feet are well cared for.

Not so long ago I was called by Ivor Shaw at nearby Thirsk Hall Farms, who asked me to trim his stock bull's feet. Whilst the trimming of the feet is a routine job, the preparation to do so can be complicated. The bull requires sedation, not because the procedure hurts, but because their feet are hard to lift. Nowadays there are mobile foot trimmers, equipped with special equipment including large restraining devices to tip bulls safely onto their sides whilst the feet are trimmed. These people travel between farms and often will trim a whole herd's feet in one visit. Without such sophisticated equipment, a vet on his own has to rely more on old-fashioned techniques. Following administration of a very strong sedative, the bull is then 'cast'.

Casting refers to the controlled throwing of an animal onto the ground by exerting pressure on its body at certain points with the help of casting ropes. The rope configuration I use is called Reuff's method, which involves a series of three loops around the body at strategic points. The sedative makes the bull wobbly, and it is then roped. The rope is pulled in the correct manner, which makes the bull roll over onto the ground, preferably onto its side in what's called 'lateral recumbency', with its feet sticking out, ready for you to work on (you don't want it to go down on its knees because you then have the added job of trying to roll it on its side).

Simple? Not when you are dealing with over a tonne of unpredictability. Indeed, as working in the field is much more hit-and-miss than when working on a patient in a veterinary clinic, I always err on the side of caution and give the patients a little bit more sedative than recommended in the data sheets to make allowances for the fact that in such cases adrenalin is coursing through my patients' veins and battling the effects of my sedative. Farmers often remark, 'By 'eck, he's fighting it, vitnary.' Once the animal is down, you get around fifteen to twenty minutes to work before the sedative starts to wear off. Each foot has two claws, so that's eight to trim. If you're lucky, you get two minutes per claw. In these situations, I've never known the clock tick away so quickly.

Risky business

On this job, Ivor and two of his colleagues were on hand to assist, because when you cast, you need to apply significant pressure to the rope to cast the bull. The bull had been injected and was getting drowsy. It was trussed up with rope, with me feeling totally in control of the situation and my helpers straining away, looking as though we were in a tug o' war contest with the bull, which was swaying and about to go down, when suddenly disaster struck as the rope snapped. The three of us hurtled backwards onto the ground. No one was hurt other than my pride as the level of adrenalin in my body turned up yet another degree.

I won't tell you what I said, but it was not professional, but neither did I feel professional at the time, having provided the rope that I had brought from home, which admittedly had been lying around for a year or two. I wasn't aware that older farm ropes had a use-by date!

Ivor sent his colleague running off to search for some rope as the seconds ticked away. Meanwhile the dazed bull continued to sway, and Ivor looked on, bemused, I felt about 2 inches tall.

Within a couple of minutes, our helper returned with a length of rope, which I tied back around the patient as quickly as I could. This time he went down. I tried to keep calm and maintain a professional aura, but underneath felt anything but. I raced between feet, feverishly clipping away, praying that the sedative kept the beast in its warm embrace for a bit longer.

Amazingly I managed to get all feet done and disentangle both sets of rope before the bull had roused enough to get grumpily to its feet.

'By 'eck,' Ivor explained when we were at a safe distance, 'that wor quicker than an F1 tyre change.'

While I managed to dodge any injury or danger by the skin of my teeth in that instance, I have noted that I've been attacked by cattle more in the last few years of my career than at any other time. I think the reason for that is the fact that farms nowadays have become bigger and much more mechanised. Small family farms where the farmers would walk among their livestock, shaking bedding up with a pitchfork and filling feeding troughs from bags of food often carried in by hand aren't common anymore, so cattle don't get used to close contact with people. Nowadays on the big farm units, cattle are often attended by somebody who drives in with a tractor and rolls big bales of bedding out. So when a human being comes along, they look at him or her and think, *What's that?*

On one farm recently I had to leap into the big metal ring feeder because a cow came for me, and it wasn't going to swerve around me at the last minute. It is not just my observation, many vets who deal with cows will say the same. For example, one of my vet colleagues broke her wrist recently while castrating a bull, due to the ferocity with which she was kicked, although in that case you could claim mitigating circumstances since there was a lot on the line as far as the bull was concerned.

Another factor is the popularity of continental breeds such as Limousin and Charolais cattle, which generally tend to be more highly strung. Perhaps they have a Gallic temperament. Becky, the wife of John Whitwell, one of the partners at Grace Lane Vets where I now work, was trampled by a continental cow recently. She was walking on a public footpath across a field with her young son and dog when a cow that was part of a herd in the field attacked her, got her down and trampled her before headbutting her. She told her son to run, which he did, as did the dog. The cow broke two of Becky's ribs, and when she put her arm up to protect her head, it kicked her again and broke that too.

Becky is a very experienced cattle vet working with them every day!

These bigger, more muscled breeds are favoured by more intensive farming enterprises in which meat is produced quickly and at quantity. They produce lean meat with less fat – the type which tends to be quite bland that you typically buy ready packaged in the supermarket. The tide seems to be turning now, however, and people are more concerned about the provenance of their food than they have been. Where does the meat come from? How far has it travelled? Has the animal been well cared for? These days many people would rather eat better quality meat in smaller amounts than previously. While a lot of the continentals are intensively reared on barley and finished off on protein pellets, there's a resurgence of interest in traditional native beef breeds like the Beef Shorthorn, which are often grass-fed and grown more slowly to maturity.

It's not just cows that pose a danger to vets of course.

Pigs can be feisty devils too, especially sows when they've got piglets with them. They are very protective and many an unfortunate farmer has been gored by the tusks of a sow looking after her piglets. You never quite know whether a pig is excited because you've got food for them or whether it denotes aggression. Pigs make a lot of noise and it's difficult to interpret what that noise means. They're hard to read and so I've always been a bit wary of them. In fact, I'd rather go into confined spaces with cattle than I would with pigs. Because on the whole, despite what I have said, the majority of cattle are slow and gentle, often lying around chewing their cud, quite content with life, while pigs seem to me much more excitable at times and difficult to read.

Even sheep, which as I explained earlier are mainly a danger to themselves, can be hazardous to deal with. We had an assistant working with us recently who was a nice chap and a good vet. A lady brought a ewe to Skeldale in the back of a trailer because she was having difficulty lambing. The vet went out to attend, and suddenly one of the nurses came running in asking for help. The vet had been knocked over by the sheep, hurt his back and couldn't continue his endeavours to bring the lambs into the world. I took over and I am pleased to report the vet made a full recovery. I laughed about it afterwards, especially upon imagining the headlines in our local newspaper, the *Darlington and Stockton Times*: 'Vet savaged by sheep!'

It is events such as these that make it important to try and stay fit as a vet, partly out of vanity I suppose and partly out of self-preservation. In large animal practice you need a level of fitness to survive. Even if you are not wrestling cattle, you are often working at your extremities trying to deliver a calf, struggling to get that leg forward or the head round. It's hard work; you get tired, especially as you get older.

The dangers faced by vets in the field create a regulatory headache in the health-and-safety conscious era in which we live. The legislation that we must work with is immense. It was decreed a few years ago when I was a partner at Skeldale that, as an employer, we should visit every farm we attend to carry out a risk assessment of the premises. When I heard that, I didn't know whether to laugh or cry. I could imagine going round some of the farms I worked on with a clipboard, marking off crushes tied together with twine and psychologically assessing sheep for any pathological traits that might make them a danger to humans, and then informing the farmer that sorry, but I can't send my vets here because your animals are too unpredictable.

In any event, often it's not the farms and the farm animals that present the biggest risk to health and safety. The closest shave I ever had was with a dog in a mechanic's yard. The dog in question was a Central Asian shepherd dog; an unusual breed to be seen around North Yorkshire and a beast of a canine. They are also known as Alabays and were bred to guard livestock. I was unfamiliar with the breed (although I became more familiar than I would have liked), but by all accounts, they are usually good-natured creatures.

There were two of these dogs, a male and female, relatively young, living with one of our local characters who owned a yard and a motor garage on the outskirts of town, in which he fixed up trucks. The unit was protected by a high boundary wall, an electric gate and, as an extra layer of protection, these two dogs, which roamed about at night discouraging anyone who might be daredevil enough to scale the already significant security perimeter.

The owner called Skeldale and requested a visit because the female was having problems with her back end.

I arrived one afternoon and buzzed the outside intercom, which crackled into life.

'Hold on a minute. I've just got to fasten the dogs,' the owner answered. In the distance I could hear deep, booming barks.

When the gates rattled open, I asked the owner, who was a big, muscular bodybuilder type of chap, whether his dogs were safe.

'The male's not to be trusted with strangers,' he said. 'He's fine with our family. The kids ride on his back, no problem, but anybody strange, I'd be worried.'

It didn't fill me with confidence. The males of the breed can grow to almost 80kg and reach seven feet tall when standing on their hind legs. He brought the bitch out, and although she was smaller, I could see what muscular and strong dogs these were. He kept a very firm hold of her, and I felt very thankful at that moment that I didn't have to examine the sharp end.

The problem was very easy to diagnose. She had a prolapsed vagina, which becomes apparent as a bitch comes into season and the vaginal wall thickens.

'The only way to treat this is to spay her after the season's finished,' I said. 'She'll be fine then.'

He agreed, and a week or so later he brought her in to the practice for the operation. Even then we were very careful with her and I insisted that he handle her until her sedative had taken effect. From then until he picked her up when she was okay to go home following a very successful surgery, I was very wary of nurses handling this hugely powerful animal.

I agreed to go and take the stitches out at his yard ten days later rather than have him bring her in to the surgery again.

So, once again I drove to his compound, buzzed the intercom and waited until the male had been put away. The gate opened, I went inside and was standing there, chatting to the owner about the bitch when suddenly I felt a massive force slam down on my back and an instant vice-like pressure on my arm. For a millisecond I was completely confused and looked at him. There was a look of horror on his face, as he yelled out, 'No! Get off!'

Then I registered the snarling noise and realised that I was being attacked.

The male had managed to get out. He had grabbed my arm and then reared up onto his hind legs, his full weight on my back and his jaws now clamped on my upper arm, trying to bring me down like a lion brings down a gazelle. The force was tremendous, as he tried to shake me like a rag doll. My survival instincts and adrenaline kicked in and I tried to pull myself free. I stood firm, knowing that if I did fall, I would be in real trouble. The dog momentarily let go of my arm and went to grab my throat. I pulled

Risky business

away from his snapping jaws as the owner, who was grappling with the beast, managed to pull him off me. The dog was barking and snarling and the man needed all his strength to drag him away.

I stood there, shaking and breathing heavily, in shock. I had been inches from having my throat ripped out. I looked down at the sleeve of my coat which was hanging in tatters. I checked myself over and breathed a sigh of relief when I realised there were only superficial cuts and bruises through my shirt, jumper and padded jacket, which had saved me. When the owner came back he was shaking too. I composed myself and continued to remove the sutures from the bitch but, to be brutally honest, I couldn't wait to get out of there.

A few minutes after I left, the owner called me.

'Are you alright, Peter?' he asked.

I knew what he meant.

'Look,' I said. 'I've never sued anybody in my life and I'm not about to start now.'

I thought for a second.

And in true Yorkshire fashion, I added, 'But I do want a new coat.'

A few days later he duly obliged.

5

Sometimes all you can do is laugh

It started like any other day, with a brew and a natter, and then a look in the daybook to see what jobs I'd be doing. It wasn't too long ago, and I was at Skeldale, getting on in years but imbued with the confidence to handle most of the things the animal kingdom could throw at me, and the wisdom to palm the job off onto someone else if I didn't feel like dealing with it, as Alf Wight did all those years ago with his crystal ball. Little was I to know that morning that later in the day I would meet my nemesis. I would meet Possum.

The entry in the daybook gave little indication of the travails to come. It simply read: *Visit Possum – cat, clip nails*. The other job options that day were a couple of bull castrations and various other, what I would call 'roughhouse', jobs. I thought back to my early training and, as I had on many occasions, I asked myself, what would Alf Wight do? I affectionately recalled Alf's use of his imaginary crystal ball in allocating work. The answer was obvious. The youngsters could get on with the physical jobs. I was going to go and see Possum. She lived with a gentleman named Robin Clough, whom I knew, so there was a chance that I might even get offered a cup of tea. *That would be lovely*, I thought to myself as I finished off my own morning cuppa.

When I mentioned to the others that I was taking the Possum job there was deathly quiet from staff working in the practice.

'Is Possum good to get on with?' I asked tentatively. There were a few mumbles and one or two smirks.

But Possum was only a cat and I'd clipped thousands of cat claws. How difficult could it be?

Indeed, if Possum was anywhere near as amenable as her owner, she'd be a. . . Well, a pussy cat.

Robin is a silver-haired retired engineer. He is very eloquent and very articulate. I know him from our local church in Bagby and he is such a good chap in every sense of the word. Sadly, his wife, Ann, died a few years ago and she adored her cats, of which they'd had several over the years. She was always the one who would ring the practice when there was a problem, for instance when one of the cats had a bit of flu or a bite that needed attention, and it was always a pleasure to visit them. They lived in a lovely sprawling country house set within beautiful walled gardens. When Ann died Robin sold it and developed the outbuildings into a very comfortable retirement home for him and Possum.

The smirks and general uneasy demeanour whenever the name Possum was mentioned gave me an inkling that perhaps things were not going to be quite as straightforward as I'd hoped.

I'll play it safe, I thought to myself, and I asked our head nurse, Rachel, to accompany me, in case I needed some help in persuading our feline patient to comply. Rachel and I got on famously, she was very practical, very useful and great to have around. She was our head nurse, and a better more useful head nurse was difficult to comprehend. She was organised, unflappable, technically brilliant, and at the same time a great person to work with, as she too possessed a dry local sense of humour.

Often cats wriggle around when they're having claws clipped, even the placid ones, and sometimes I found it helpful to wrap them in a blanket with the leg which required attention protruding. I mentioned this to Rachel, and along with the little clippers, she found a nice big bath towel that we could use to swaddle Possum.

When we arrived, Robin met us at the door.

'How lovely to see you,' he said. 'It's very kind of you to come. Possum is waiting for you upstairs.'

I momentarily wondered why Robin hadn't brought Possum down to us.

'Is she good to get on with, Robin?' I asked.

He looked sheepish.

'Oh, she has her moments, Peter,' he said. 'She can be a little bit feisty sometimes but I'm sure she'll be absolutely fine.'

I wasn't fully reassured, and, along with Rachel, Robin took us up the stairs and into the master bedroom. Robin pointed to the dressing table.

'She's under there,' he said.

'Hello, Possum,' I said reassuringly, and bent down to look at her.

She looked back at me, and I'll never forget those menacing, threatening eyes. They were like the eyes of the devil, black as the darkest night. I shivered and turned to Rachel.

'I think we might need that towel,' I muttered.

I attempted to coax Possum out with some friendly words of encouragement and the offer of some treats. She was defiant and just sat there, glaring at me.

'I'm not so sure about this, Robin,' I said.

He excused himself.

'I'll just be downstairs if you need me,' he said as he backed out of the door.

I decided that the best way to approach Possum was from the side of the table, where there was enough room to bend down and get hold of her. I made my move very slowly and got within six inches of her. I reached out my hand when suddenly her eyes lit up and she bared her teeth. She hissed and spat and her foot came at my hand with claws extended quicker than a punch from Muhammad Ali. I only just managed to pull my hand back in time before it was shredded.

'Bloody hell!' I exclaimed. I reached back to Rachel to get the towel, and as I turned, Possum shot out from under the dressing table and dashed into another room where she took refuge under a bed.

Rachel and I set off in pursuit and I crouched down to look under the valance to see what we were dealing with. From a dark corner those eyes glinted, and a low growl reverberated through the air.

'There's no way I'm putting my arm under there,' I told Rachel. 'We'll need something to nudge her out with.'

We found Robin's old walking stick and I lay on my belly to try and gently poke Possum. The tactic worked. The cat moved but scarpered out from under the bed and then dashed under a wardrobe.

I got the impression this was just a game for Possum. She knew who was in control and I was a toy to be played with. Rachel was smiling. It was turning into a farce.

'Right,' I determined, 'here's what we are going to do. We'll block off the exit routes so she can only escape in one direction, and when she does, we'll throw the towel over her.'

The plan worked, sort of.

Using the walking stick again, I got Possum to come out from under the wardrobe and Rachel threw the towel on her. I tried to get a grip on the thrashing bundle but there were claws going everywhere, and within two seconds the towel was left in a heap on the floor and Possum had once again departed.

I knew we were defeated. There was no way now an agitated Possum was going to let us get anywhere near her.

'This isn't going to work,' I sighed. 'We're going to have to come back and bring reinforcements. This is Possum one, Peter nil. We'll come back with a sedative.'

Despairingly, I went down to see Robin.

'We failed,' I admitted. 'Possum is a bit of a handful.'

'Well,' he said as he lowered his newspaper, 'she can be a little bit difficult sometimes. She doesn't really like me either.'

He explained that in the evening Possum would come into the house.

'But she can't stand me, so she goes and sits in another room on her own,' he said.

He explained that recently some friends came round, and they sat down and had a cup of tea and Possum took an interest in the wife.

'She was obviously very good with cats, this lady,' recounted Robin. 'Possum jumped up onto her knee and was letting her stroke her. It was quite remarkable. Anyway, Possum then jumped down again and the husband thought he would have a go. He bent down to pick Possum up and put her on his knee.

'Within thirty seconds I was striding into the kitchen for the first-aid box.'

With a better picture of what I was dealing with, I arranged to come back another day with a sedative and asked Robin if he

Sometimes all you can do is laugh

could starve Possum before we came, as sedatives can sometimes induce vomiting.

A few days later, Rachel and I were back again, properly equipped with a sedative, towels, a big blanket, heavy leather gauntlets, nail clippers and a crush cage, which is like a metal cat carrier with a moveable partition inside that can be positioned using external arms. My plan was to get Possum in the cage, push her against the side using the partition and then inject her with a sedative.

Once again Robin showed us in and once again Possum was in her usual position under the dressing table, looking at us with hate-filled eyes. She obviously recognised me because she launched into a volley of feline abuse which I'm sure was akin to barracks language.

'You're not going to win this time,' I told her.

We sealed off all escape exits around the table and shut the door. Possum, sensing that it was round two, continued with her abuse. She was up for a fight. I started towards her, and she hissed and made a move. As she bolted from under the table, I threw the blanket over her like a net, and this time it was too big for her to get out from under. That gave us a chance. I got on top of the blanket and quickly felt the angry, writhing shape underneath. I found her neck and grabbed the scruff through the material, which is politically incorrect, but this was a needs-must situation. I managed to pick her up and position her over the top of the cage, opened it up, dropped her in and shut it.

Possum was neutralised! I felt victorious. The language coming from her was indescribable. She was hissing and spitting like a banshee. She was a wild thing. *This is the cat from hell*, I thought to myself.

With her in the cage and under control, I was able to press her against the side and sedate her, and then have a proper look at her. What I discovered gave a clue as to why she was so bad tempered.

When a cat sharpens its claws on furniture or on a tree, it is removing dead fibres, which shale off, keeping the claws sharp and shortened. Sometimes older cats who don't go out as much don't sharpen their nails enough and the claws grow thick and curl round. This had happened to Possum and her claws were growing into her pads.

This wouldn't have done much for her temper, but unless you got up close and personal to Possum, you'd never know, and because Possum didn't let Robin near her, he couldn't see that this was happening.

With Possum now fast asleep, I took her out of the cage and started work on her claws while Rachel watched carefully for signs that the sedation was stable and not wearing off. There was a lot to cut back, and when I'd finished there were massive amounts of nail clippings all over the floor.

Once we'd cleared up and taken our equipment outside, I gave Possum the antidote to the anaesthetic, which felt a bit like lighting a firework. We knew to stand well clear.

We watched to make sure she came round satisfactorily. She was groggy and bad tempered, so we knew she was okay.

I went down to see Robin who was sitting reading his newspaper again unperturbed by the screeching and hissing he'd heard.

'Mission accomplished, Robin,' I said proudly.

'Thank you so much. I'm so appreciative and I'm sure Possum will be as well. I can't thank you enough for coming to do it,' he said. 'I'm grateful I didn't have to attempt it.'

Sometimes all you can do is laugh

We had a cup of tea with Robin, and before I left, I went back upstairs, tiptoed to open the door, looked around the corner, and saw Possum once again sitting under the dressing table, glaring out with those eyes, filled with hate. I've never been so glad to see a patient controlled by sedation in all my life.

A couple of years later I saw Robin in church, and he explained that Possum's nails were starting to cause a problem again.

He spoke apologetically.

'Do you mind calling round to see her?' he asked.

'I'll look forward to it,' I replied, laughing, 'but I think we should sedate her from the start.'

Thankfully, part two of Possum vs Peter was not as eventful. By that stage Possum was older and a little more frail so we didn't have quite the same battle, but by God, the old Possum was still there alive and kicking and hissing like a demon.

And while Possum was a handful, I'd gladly take my chances with her than tackle one of the more unusual patients I was called to see a while later.

Peter Jolly's Circus was one of the last two travelling circuses to use big cats in its act before wild animals were banned in circuses in 2019. The traditional travelling circus was established fifty years ago and had camels, zebras, horses, ponies, dogs, ducks, pigeons and snakes amongst other animals. Each year the circus travelled around the country from location to location where they pitched the big top and put on their show.

The circus ran through Mr Jolly's blood, and while animal welfare campaigners had long highlighted the issue of using performing animals, calling it cruel and inhumane, he cared for his animals and was licenced by the government to keep wild ones. Under the terms of the licence, he required three Defra (The

Department for Environment, Food and Rural Affairs) inspections a year and four vet inspections to make sure that the animals were being cared for. The purpose of each inspection was to check that the animals were properly fed and watered, that their environment was up to Defra standards and, just as importantly, that their behavioural needs were being catered for.

The circus was performing near Thirsk, and Mr Jolly came to the Skeldale practice as one of his quarterly inspections was due.

He was an avuncular man, good-humoured, thoughtful and humble. No matter what your views on whether circuses were wrong or right, I could tell he had a good heart and took the welfare of his animals seriously. He'd been born into circus life and knew nothing else. Yet he was part of a dying breed, and it must have been obvious to him at that time that the clock was ticking down on his way of life and public opinion was turning against it. Indeed, within a few years of our meeting, his animal troupe was disbanded. He seemed like a man with a weight on his shoulders. It was very obvious he wanted to do the best for his animals and his people. He asked me if I would do the scheduled inspection. At first, I was uncertain.

At that stage in my career, I did a lot of what we call clipboard work for the local authority, such as riding school, boarding and breeding establishment inspections, and this was a clipboard job, albeit with more exotic animals, which concerned me.

'Are there any wild or large game animals there?' I asked. 'As I'm not really experienced at handling them.'

Peter reassured me.

'There are,' he said, 'but you won't need to handle them, and the handlers will be there. It won't be a problem at all.'

'I've never liked snakes,' I explained.

'I'll be honest, we have half a dozen snakes, but you won't have to go in with them. You just need to look at them, make sure they're healthy and looked after properly,' he said.

He also explained that there was a fox called Samantha, a Bactrian camel, and an Ankole bull.

When I realised that I didn't have to examine any of the menagerie but purely inspect their behaviour and environment instead, I agreed. Peter explained that when the circus wasn't travelling it was based in Shropshire, where they used a vet I knew, a gentleman named Lloyd Jones who qualified from Liverpool a few years after me and who I had occasionally played football with in the past, when we were both younger and fitter. Our profession is quite small compared with others so it was lovely to be able to give Lloyd a call that evening, catch up on old times and ensure there would be no nasty surprises for me at the circus.

'There's nothing ominous there, Peter,' he told me. 'Even for a mixed practice vet it should be no problem.'

Lloyd is a level-headed, sensible vet and if he said it was fine, then that'll do for me, I thought.

A few days later I arrived at the circus, clipboard in hand, and with the necessary forms, and I've got to admit, Peter's husbandry was good. All the animals were well cared for, and even though the massive pythons were not my cup of tea, I could see all their required feeding programmes, environmental requirements and behavioural needs were met; also, his record keeping was meticulous.

It was a simple tick-box exercise, and I enjoyed being there. I filled in the paperwork, which was sent off, and came away relieved that the job wasn't as onerous as I'd initially feared.

Three months later the circus was back in Thirsk and the inspection was due again. Once more, Peter came to see me and this time I had no reservations about carrying out the work. I got the paperwork that was required, took my clipboard, and went back out to visit as staff were busily erecting the big top for the show. I started to carry out the inspection, feeling quite confident.

And then one of the handlers sidled up to me.

'Er, Peter, the tiger's lame, would you mind having a look at her, please?' he asked.

I looked at him and blinked. Tiger! I thought, *This wasn't in the script. This wasn't supposed to happen.*

As a vet I'd been trained to never turn down the opportunity to help an animal in need, nor was it in my nature. But I'd also never been asked to examine an apex predator. My mind was in turmoil as I tried to work out how I could extricate myself from the situation with professional pride intact. I didn't want to look like a coward, but how the hell was I supposed to examine a tiger? I tried to reason with myself. They're just big cats, right? They have the same physiology as a common moggy, only bigger and more deadly. And then I thought of Possum.

Peter, I told myself, you fought Possum, the deadliest cat in North Yorkshire. You fought Possum and you prevailed. If you can face Possum, surely you can take a quick look at a lame, tame tiger.

'Okay,' I said meekly to the handler, my hands trembling, clutching a clipboard which would have been useless had I needed it to defend myself.

The walk across to the tiger's cage felt like the walk of a condemned man to the execution chamber. The handler looked at me and could see I was a paler shade of white and visibly shaking.

'Are you alright?' he asked.

'Fine,' I lied. And then: 'How tame is the tiger, exactly?'

The handler started to laugh.

'You don't think I'd let you get in with her, do you? I only want you to have a look through the bars.'

A tsunami of relief swept over me, and I tried not to look like a pillock, even though I felt like one.

'Of course not,' I bluffed.

The tiger was a magnificent creature, and, from a safe distance, I studied her carefully as she moved. Sadly, I could tell that there was something amiss. It was only a hunch and nothing more, but I feared the worst. She had mild muscle atrophy in her upper forelimb. I suspected bone cancer.

This could be something nasty, I thought to myself.

Bone cancer can be very aggressive, and inoperable, and it often metastasises, which means it spreads to other parts of the body.

'I don't know for definite without a proper examination, but I think it could be something serious,' I explained. 'I think you may have to take her to the University of Liverpool or somewhere on your way home where they've got the facilities to handle her, anaesthetise her and examine her properly.'

The handler was grateful for my opinion, and I left him with some painkillers which we use on dogs and cats to put in her food.

I could tell how concerned he was. Whether you agree with circuses or not, it was very clear that the people looked after their animals well and cared for them as you would expect from animal lovers who live and work with animals day in, day out. Going back in time, people didn't go abroad on holiday, they went to places like Scarborough, Blackpool or Eastbourne and they didn't get a chance to see all these wonderful exotic creatures unless they were in circuses or zoos. Nowadays as people travel the world, the educational value of these establishments, especially zoos, has diminished and the main purpose of them has become for conservation work.

I asked the handler to let me know what happened, and a few weeks later I was leafing through the daybook and saw a message from Jolly's Circus. The tiger had been taken somewhere in Manchester which had the required handling facilities. She was X-rayed, and sadly she did have bone cancer and had to be put to sleep.

Whilst I was fortunate enough on that occasion not to have got too up-close-and-personal with a tiger, I have had plenty of experience handling exotics, as we call them.

One recent case involved Dave, the emu chick who came to Skeldale with an ulcerated eye and facial injuries. Dave belonged to Steve, a Thirsk resident who kept other exotic birds and had named his chick after his friend who had sadly recently passed away.

Dave, the emu, had been attacked by a dog. He was looking very sorry for himself when Steve brought him in, in a shopping basket. I examined him and saw that a tooth had punctured the skin on his face. The real concern was the eye, which had suffered a lot of trauma and was crusted over with a layer of crud and debris which I carefully removed. It was touch-and-go whether Dave's eyelid and eye could be saved. I gave Steve drops to apply several times a day to try and save it.

An ulcerated eye can go one of two ways. It can either heal or the ulcer can deepen and rupture. It's a very painful process as well, which is why poor Dave was also put on painkillers.

Steve was very attached to his little mate and was distressed by the whole episode. He had sat up with Dave all night after the attack, and explained that the chick had brightened up by the time he got to the surgery. He was beating himself up and believed he shouldn't have allowed the dogs a chance to get to Dave.

'These things happen,' I told him. 'You can't blame yourself.'

Thankfully, Dave did well, and we were able to save his eye.

Sometimes all you can do is laugh

I happened upon one of Steve's feathered friends three years later in bizarre circumstances one summer after a wonderful day out at the annual Thirsk Picnic in the Park. The festival is one of the highlights of the town's social calendar and involves live music, food stalls, entertainment and often a few pints of Yorkshire's finest Black Sheep ale. The year in question I had appeared on the stage with the local celebrities Nick Hancock and Will Smith from Stray FM, a radio station based in Harrogate. They were compering the event. We'd had a bit of a chat and drawn a raffle, and after I'd done my bit, I relaxed with my wife, Lin, and our friends Stephen and Jeanette. Together we had a good time and a really good knees-up. All in all, it was a lovely day and evening, and I was just reflecting with Lin how lovely it was to be part of such a close-knit community as we were driving back through Bagby on our way home, and were about fifty yards from Steve's property, situated on the main street through the village, when something strange happened. It was around midnight and getting dark, and as we passed the entrance of a cul-de-sac called Sandown Close, two older teenage girls walked into the road and frantically flagged us down.

'Can you help us? We've just seen an ostrich,' they said.

Well, I'd had a drop to drink, and I thought these girls had obviously been on the bottle too. Then I realised where we were and remembered Steve.

'Stop the car, Lin. I might have some work to do,' I said comically.

She parked up and we got out of the car and looked down the cul-de-sac. Sure enough, bathed in orange streetlight, stood a huge, shaggy bird with a long neck. It looked at us, and we looked at it.

I walked a bit closer and the bird, which I thought was an emu but later learned was a rhea, turned around and casually strutted into a garden.

'We can't just leave it,' said Lin. And I agreed. But I was in no fit state to wrestle it on my own and what would I do with it anyway?

Luckily, my Skeldale partner Tim lived very close by and I could see the light was still on in his front room, so I ran over and knocked on his door. Tim was one of the nicest blokes you could wish to meet and one of the best vets I ever knew. He was also at Liverpool University, qualifying two years behind me, and came to work at Kirkgate in 1984. We came up through the ranks together and Tim joined me in the partnership in 1990 before retiring in 2000. Tim was a very quiet man, always shying away from any limelight but always dependable. You could literally trust him with your life.

He answered the door.

'It's a funny time of night for a social call. Do you know what time it is?' he asked with a raised brow. 'I was just going to bed.'

'There's a bloody great emu wandering around in the road opposite,' I said.

He sighed. 'That'll be one of Steve's rheas. I'm bloody sick of putting those things back. Hang on a minute, I'll go and get one of my socks and the wheelbarrow.'

It transpired that Steve's rheas made a habit of breaking out and Tim, as the nearest animal expert, was often tasked with getting them back in their enclosure, which was in Steve's back garden. It was such a common occurrence that Tim had a well-practised 'rhea wrestling routine'.

I went back over the road where Lin was keeping an eye out to make sure the bird remained in the garden it had retreated to, and a few minutes later Tim joined us with his wheelbarrow and his sock.

The garden belonged to the retired publican of the Forresters Arms in Kilburn, Peter Cousins, whom I'd known for many years,

Sometimes all you can do is laugh

having frequented his excellent establishment on numerous occasions. He was very good at diplomatically persuading customers to leave at the end of the night but his expertise did not extend to removing big birds from his garden. I knocked on his door. He answered in his dressing gown and looked a little bleary eyed. He'd obviously been asleep.

'I'm sorry to bother you, Peter,' I said. 'Some girls flagged me down because they've seen this rhea in the Close, and I'm pretty sure it's strutted into your garden. Do you mind us checking to see if it's still there, please?'

He walked off and came back a few seconds later to confirm that yes, there was a flipping great bird trampling his begonias.

'Tim's here with his sock and a wheelbarrow, which he assures me are the tools needed for the job, and we'll remove it for you and take it back home if you would allow us,' I said.

'Help yourself. You can use the side gate. But if you don't mind, I'm going back to bed.'

He shut the door and I heard it lock. He wanted no part of the debacle and I couldn't blame him.

Tim and I stalked up the side path and through the gate, trying to remain silent so as not to startle the rhea. The only sounds were my stifled giggles and the squeak-squeak-squeak of Tim's wheelbarrow. The bird eyed us suspiciously.

'You grab it around the chest, I'll put the sock over its head, and we'll tip it into the barrow and wheel it back round to Steve's,' explained Tim.

The bird was used to humans and allowed us to get close enough to execute the plan.

I lunged and got it in a bear hug. It made a startled sound and stamped its legs. Tim pulled the sock expertly over its head, which seemed to pacify it, and then he tipped the wheelbarrow on its side, at which point I pushed it into the barrow's cradle and Tim then righted it. It was over in a second and the rhea was on its side in the wheelbarrow, passively resigned to having been caught. As a precaution I held it down in place. It struggled a bit but it knew the game was up. Tim pushed it back out of Peter's garden, past his bedroom window, which was now in total darkness, and down the road to Steve's house. We resolved not to wake another resident and let ourselves into Steve's back garden, where we found an empty pen that we assumed belonged to our captive. We unloaded the bird into the pen, took the sock off, locked the gate after us and left the bird strutting about, ruffling its feathers with nothing hurt, other than its pride. Tim went back to bed muttering about how bloody sick he was of these rheas, and Lin and I got back in the car and drove off home with me wondering if I'd just had a weird dream. When I realised it had really happened, I don't know if it was the spectacle we had just witnessed or the effect of the alcohol still present in my system, or a combination of both, but I started to laugh uncontrollably.

6

Sad cases

The phone trilled on Joan's desk; she reached over, picked it up and my heart sank when I heard her reply to the caller.

'Again, Mr Harding?' She frowned. 'Yes, of course. I'll let him know.'

She replaced the receiver and looked over at me with a mixture of concern and pity.

'That was Ken Harding,' she said. 'He needs you up there. It's happening again.'

I'd not been long back in Thirsk and had just finished morning surgery, which had been uneventful. There had been a cat with an abscess to attend to. It was a particularly placid tortoiseshell female which had an infected wound in a rather unfortunate place on her back end. She was very good natured and allowed me to drain the wound without putting up too much of a struggle. Abscesses were one of the most common conditions we see in cats on account of their propensity to fight and the number of horrible bacteria they carry in their mouths. Indeed, later in my career I knew a woman who suffered nerve damage and hand paralysis because of an infection from a cat bite. As the professional in the consulting room, if a cat patient bit its owner, I would be deemed responsible and would be required to direct the owner to go to the doctors and have the injury attended to. Failure to do so would be classed as negligence on my part. This was just one of the nuggets of regulatory information I was learning. In fact, many of our nurses at Skeldale over the years have required hospital treatment for cat bites.

But thankfully, that morning's patient was compliant. The wound on its backside was a puncture, caused by a rival's tooth or claw, which had sealed over to create a perfect closed environment for bacteria to multiply.

'Not much of a scrapper this one, eh?' I said to the owner as I cleaned up the wound.

'No, she's not, how can you tell?' she asked.

'The wound is on her back end. She was running away.'

With the cat dealt with, there were a few vaccinations to administer and a lame red setter to attend, together with an off-colour tortoise. By the time Mr Harding phoned, it had been an unremarkable morning and I was looking forward to a sit-down and some lunch. The call changed all that.

Mr Harding's woes were an ongoing saga that was becoming a tragedy. Old Ken had a farm bordering the North York Moors and was a man of simplicity and endeavour. His farm was run like his life, slowly, purposefully and according to the rhythm of the seasons. He was a man of few words who lived in a beautiful spot in the hills where his collection of ramshackle moss-covered stone outbuildings looked like they had grown from the ground up and were as much a part of the landscape as the trees.

Ken had a dairy herd and around fifteen young heifers, which are immature cows that have never had a calf before. The heifers were Friesians, which are lean-framed and bred to produce milk. They were petite and skittish. Nine months previously Ken had made a disastrous decision that was now coming back to haunt him, and me. To maximise the yield from his herd he decided to put a Limousin bull onto the heifers, which was a big, highly-muscled continental animal. By his reckoning, the resulting calves would grow bigger, thereby maximising the value of the calves that he would sell on at market.

What Ken hadn't foreseen was that the calves produced by this union were far too big to be born naturally. Initially, Ken had tried to deliver the first few himself, until he realised there was a pattern emerging and began phoning Kirkgate for help on a regular basis. Only a few of the pregnant heifers managed to calve naturally, and those that did almost died in the process due to the trauma. Others had sadly died. Most required delivery by caesarean section, and in the worst cases, in my opinion, the calves had died inside their mothers during birth.

I used to dread the phone calls, some of which occurred in the middle of the night when I was on call. It was an utter disaster. In Ken's defence, he had no idea this was going to happen, and as the death toll started to rise, I could tell that even this quiet and somewhat cynical farmer was mortified by the situation and horrified at the suffering these young heifers were going through.

When I arrived at the farm that afternoon it was my fifth visit that month and Ken looked dejected. It was a late-spring day and the weather was glorious, but the sunshine and clear blue skies did nothing to lift our moods. There was a very dark cloud hanging over Ken.

'It's another one, I'm afraid,' he said to me as he trudged into the cowshed fearing another salvage job. I followed and looked sadly at the struggling heifer standing in the shade at the far end of the building. She was straining hard, with shallow breathing and glazed eyes. There was an air of hopelessness about her and I could see she was already looking exhausted.

We didn't need to speak but I asked Ken anyway.

'Had a go yourself?'

He shook his head.

'Not this time.'

I began my examination, but I knew what I'd find.

When examining a cow in labour, the vet feels for the position of the calf. When you have a multiple birth, this can present a challenge as, in the tight confines of a uterus, you must feel for legs and heads and work out which way round they all are and what body part belongs to which calf. Sometimes it can be deceiving. You feel two legs facing forward and assume they both belong to the same calf, when in fact one belongs to one and the other to the second sibling jostling behind but racing to be born first. In such cases you must repel the one behind and get the one in front in the correct position to be born. In an ideal world there will be two front legs and a head belonging to the same calf, all facing towards the rear of the cow in the birth canal. In that situation all a vet needs to do to help the mother along is give a pull on the legs. If the calf is in the wrong position, or if there are two calves in a bit of a jumble, some careful manipulation is required.

The same rules and strategies apply whether it be a calf, a puppy, or a lamb. If you put your hand in and there's just a tail and no legs, this indicates that both back legs are facing forward towards the mother's head, and this can be quite tricky because you've got to get both hind legs facing towards the rear end of the mother to give you the opportunity of pulling the calf out backwards.

Sad cases

With Ken's heifer I could feel into the uterus and only felt the rump of the calf. Which meant it was out of position. This is called a breach presentation and in such cases it is impossible for the calf to be born naturally without manipulation. But when I stretched further to gauge its dimensions, it was clear that it was far too big to be born through the birth canal. My spirits lifted slightly when I felt it move. At least it was alive.

I withdrew my arm and told Ken what I'd discovered.

'The good news is that it's still alive, the bad news is it'll have to be another caesarean section,' I explained.

Ken nodded.

'Right you are,' he muttered in a resigned manner.

The calf had a fighting chance but with the mother clearly exhausted and in distress I had to move fast.

Being a vet is about making decisions, and throughout my career I have constantly questioned whether I've made the right ones. Often, they are life-and-death decisions, made quickly. All you can do is base your actions on training and experience. In this case I made the right decision, and after administering a local anaesthetic and cutting into the flank of the mother, I was able to pull the calf out, with Ken's help.

It flopped onto the straw on the floor in a messy heap, and as I started to sew up the cow's uterus, Ken rubbed the new-born vigorously until I heard it make a choking bleat when it took its first gulp of air. As I looked round I saw the calf raise and shake its head to announce its arrival in the world.

Relief washed over me, and I offered a silent prayer of thanks.

I couldn't be angry with Ken. He'd made an honest mistake those nine months ago for which he was being severely punished. A lot of Yorkshire farmers will not show their feelings, but as Ken knelt over the new-born, gently rubbing it now, I could see his eyes moisten and could tell he was hurting from what he'd done and was frustrated that he couldn't rectify it. He just had to accept what had happened and make the best of a bad job.

He encouraged the calf gently to the mother, who by now was showing signs of a new lease of life, chewing absent-mindedly on some hay as if nothing had happened. Animals truly are the most remarkable beings. She eyed the mega-baby standing in front of her, bent down, sniffed it and started to lick it.

'Job's a good 'un,' said Ken.

'Aye,' I answered, feeling a bit teary myself.

'I'm not going to make this mistake again,' he said. It was one of the longest conversations we ever had. Ken, I believed, had accepted by that point that he was probably better on the arable side of farming than he was as a stockman.

Life and death are constant companions in the veterinary world. They ebb and flow, and if you get home at the end of a shift having seen more life than death, you've had a relatively good day. Sometimes death happens naturally, and we help owners see their beloved companions pass away peacefully at the end of long and well-lived life; other times it happens tragically and suddenly, or because of an illness. Sometimes there are no explanations, and an animal dies for no apparent reason. I recall one case going back in time at Skeldale when a dog was brought in that couldn't stop vomiting. He was X-rayed, I took blood samples and did every test possible. I tried all I could, but he died. I never knew why. I could never get to the bottom of it, and as a vet, not knowing the answer can be soul-destroying.

One of the first lessons you learn when you become a vet is that you should never take it personally, but you do. We can't help

Sad cases

but care because we're humans and we see the relationships that develop between owners and their pets every single day, and we also see the pain when the bonds of love they share break.

I remember one elderly chap's dog I went to visit one night after surgery. He was living on his own, a widower, his wife long since passed, his children grown and moved away. His only companion was his old Staffordshire bull terrier. She was barrel-chested, slow on her feet and grey-whiskered, but the old man adored her, and she adored her owner, who was very poorly and practically housebound. The two of them were living out their final days together.

The man had called and requested a visit because he was too infirm to get to the surgery himself. He was worried about the dog because that morning he had awoken and seen she was in considerable discomfort. She was uncharacteristically off her food and sat on her bed all day, whimpering occasionally. I offered to go and check after work because I didn't want to leave her until morning if there was something I could do sooner rather than later to solve the problem.

The old chap was frail and took a while to answer the door. Worry was etched across his face as he led me to the kitchen where the dog was lying on her bed. She looked up with sad eyes. She couldn't stand, the man explained, and had been getting worse throughout the day. I knelt and palpated her abdomen. She whimpered loudly.

I knew what the problem was, and the prognosis was not good. I could feel a very large mid-abdominal mass, which was almost certainly a splenic tumour. The spleen is one organ that can be removed, but sometimes, if they are not picked up in time, such splenic masses can rupture and the animal dies, sometimes in minutes, as they bleed internally. I could feel the mass and I could tell also that her abdomen was full of fluid, which was almost certainly blood. It was hopeless. The only kind option was to put her to sleep. I explained this to the man gently and I could see his frail frame crumple.

'I'll put the kettle on. Let's have a cup of tea,' I said.

I made us both a brew and we sat and chatted for almost an hour while I let the man get used to the sad reality that he was going to lose his best friend. When the time was right, I let him say his goodbyes and I put her to sleep, while he stroked her head, tears running down his cheeks.

The following day I told one of my colleagues what had happened.

'That poor old chap's world just caved in and I'm worried about him,' I said. 'I don't think he'll live much longer.'

About six weeks later our account keeper happened to mention that the bill for visiting the old man and his beloved dog had not been paid. When I investigated, I discovered that the man had died two days after his dog. I think he just gave up.

The most shocking and tragic event I ever witnessed during my time as a vet, however, happened a few years ago in Skeldale and is indelibly etched on my memory.

Sarah and James were a couple I'd known for many years. They were lovely people and had a smallholding at the foot of the Hambleton Hills not too far from Thirsk. Sarah was the local commissioner of the Pony Club and her life revolved around horses and ponies. She was a really energetic, get-up-and-go woman who lived life to the full and brought a sense of warmth and fun everywhere she went. Her husband, James, was the same. They both had lots of interests and were busy, intelligent people, who were pillars of the community. They also loved their Labradors and had several litters over the years, which I attended with great pleasure.

Sad cases

One of the Labradors, who I had attended throughout, was now in the twilight of her life and had lost her zest for living. Sarah and James had observed that her quality of life had recently diminished. She was arthritic, in pain, finding it hard to get up and down, and struggling with life generally. Sarah and James, ever the pragmatists, realised that it had reached the point where it was time to say goodbye, and so they made an appointment one morning to bring her in and do the compassionate thing.

Any pet owner who has been through this understands what a difficult decision it is. We'd like our pets to live forever, of course, but they don't, and often, the kindest thing an owner can do is to recognise the time is right to call an end to the animal's suffering at the end of their life.

In these situations, whenever I can, I arrange for the owners to bring their pets in at the end of surgery when the practice is quiet. People don't want to come and sit in the waiting room queuing up to be seen, and in their situation neither would I. It is an emotional and difficult time.

Sarah and James arrived late morning with their dog, which they carried into the consulting room. I had a quick look at her and I agreed that the quality of her life didn't warrant continuing. I assured them that they had made the right decision and they were doing the correct thing. Conversely, there have been numerous times when in the same position I have told owners the time is not yet right, and they have returned home again.

What happened next is so clear in my mind that I remember it as if it were yesterday. I can remember the exact position everyone was in. The dog was on the floor lying on her blanket, I was kneeling with her. James was standing in front of me, and Sarah was at my left-hand side, stroking the old girl as I prepared the injection of pentobarbital. I asked a nurse to help me raise a vein. Everyone was quiet. It was a solemn time as the couple were losing their beloved and loyal companion who meant a lot to them. The only sound was Sarah, whispering a goodbye.

The room fell silent as I injected the pentobarbital. As it began to take effect and the dog's breathing slowed, I felt something slump against my left shoulder and was then aware of someone on the floor by my side. I looked over. It was Sarah. She wasn't moving and the colour had drained from her face. I thought she had fainted. The dog had stopped breathing, and I turned to Sarah and shook her, then turned her on her side. She was completely motionless. James stood there in shock.

I can't remember anyone speaking but we must have. Everything seemed to speed up. Sarah's face turned grey. I checked for a heartbeat and pulse, which was weak and intermittent, before fading out. She wasn't breathing.

Skeldale was next door to a St John's Ambulance station, so I asked the nurse to run and see if there was anyone who could help while I called 999. I then started administering CPR. After what seemed like an eternity but was probably only a few minutes, two paramedics arrived and managed to stabilise Sarah's heart. They wired her up to an ECG. It didn't appear that she'd had a heart attack.

Her heart stopped again, and they continued their best endeavours, managing to restart it once more. The ambulance team then arrived. They felt that Sarah was sufficiently stable for them to take her to hospital. James, who was in a daze, went with her, while their dearly beloved companion, motionless and completely forgotten by us all, was left on the consulting room floor.

Sarah's heart stopped again on the way to hospital, and they couldn't resuscitate her. She died in the ambulance with James by her side. It later transpired that she'd suffered a brain haemorrhage.

Everyone in the practice was in complete shock for several days. I went home in tears that night. How could it have happened? There was no logic to it. James was a widower. He came in with his wife and a beloved pet and went home without either of them. It was the saddest day I can remember, and it altered my outlook on life somewhat. We worry about the small things going on in our lives, we get frustrated when things don't go our way, or when things take longer than we expect. We worry about money, possessions, and these things then just pale into complete insignificance when you witness just how fragile human life is and how vulnerable we are. Sarah was sixty-three. She shouldn't have died.

7

Miracles can happen

The black Labrador limping towards me looked up hopefully and wagged her tail. I could tell she was poorly. She was panting and lethargic and looked very sorry for herself, but she still had a faint sparkle in her eyes. If she could talk, she would have been saying: 'I'm okay, I'm just a bit under the weather.'

Her owner had brought her in to Skeldale several days previously with a limp and a small lump on her front leg. The owner lived at the top of Sutton Bank on the edge of the North York Moors, and she'd been out with her two-year-old dog doing something called beating.

Some folks do not agree with it but in the countryside, shooting is a popular activity that employs a lot of people and contributes to a significant percentage of the rural economy. Beaters and their dogs go ahead of the guns and beat the bushes and cover where the pheasants, partridges and ducks shelter. The birds take flight for the shooters to target. In my opinion the social element is the most important thing for a lot of people who take part in shooting, and they enjoy getting dressed up in their regalia and spending time with their mates. For many of them though, as I have witnessed, can't wait to get in the pub afterwards. Others derive more pleasure from beating than shooting. Their dogs are trained to retrieve quarry, and they get to spend time exercising outdoors with their beloved companions, working together as a team.

On the dog in question's first visit, the limb was checked over and it was thought she'd had a bump on a rock as there was a slight swelling but nothing else to see.

But several days later her condition deteriorated, and she was back at Skeldale when I was the vet on duty.

The owner was worried.

'She's just not herself. She's carrying the leg; it's swollen and it's bleeding. She's off her food and very depressed,' the owner explained.

I knelt and patted the dog on her head. She looked at me again with doe-eyed innocence. I lifted her leg carefully to take a closer look and what I saw concerned me. The leg was much more swollen. What had previously been a small lump had now expanded to become a large soft swelling that extended up the leg. Underneath the hair I could see the skin was bruised purple and deep red. At the centre of the swelling, where the initial injury would have been, the skin was punctured and weeping watery blood.

I only had to touch the leg slightly and she pulled it away quickly and yelped.

I recognised the symptoms.

'She's been bitten by a snake,' I said to the owner.

In the UK we have one venomous snake, which is the adder, and they are not particularly common but there happen to be quite a lot of them on the North York Moors. They are shy creatures by nature and are not aggressive but will defend themselves if they feel threatened. I have seen several snake bite injuries over the years, generally from spring through to summer and into early autumn, although one year I dealt with one on Boxing Day, when a boisterous patient had obviously disturbed a hibernating snake.

The seriousness of the bite depends on how much venom enters the bloodstream and how quickly the bite is treated. If the snake catches a blood vessel, for example, the effects will be worse – and can even be fatal – than if it's just a bite on an extremity where the venom often remains localised. A majority will get better on their own. If, however, the venom has time to circulate in the system, it becomes a more complex case which can lead to liver and kidney failure and death. After several days post-bite, antivenom injections become ineffective.

This was the situation I found myself in. Although we carried stocks of antivenom at the practice, it would have been useless. I thought for a moment and explained to the owner that we would have to admit her and keep her at the practice where we could provide supportive treatment.

'We'll look after her,' I promised, 'but this could be a difficult few days for her. She's still wagging her tail, and that's a good sign, but she's going to have to fight this herself and her condition will worsen.'

The lady nodded and bent down to say her goodbyes.

'She's in good hands,' I tried to reassure her.

We made the dog as comfortable as we could and got her in a kennel to immobilise her, because the calmer and stiller she was, the less chance the venom had to disperse further round her body. We began a treatment programme which included painkillers, antibiotics and a supportive intravenous drip. Over the next few hours, the poor thing began looking increasingly miserable. She was breathing hard and looked increasingly depressed. My optimism was evaporating, but whenever someone gave her a bit of attention there was still that faint wag of her tail, which, over the coming days, symbolised hope. Because things did become much worse.

Over the next twenty-four hours her breathing became more laboured and the skin damage spread. The skin around the site of the bite, which was bruised and bloody, began to turn black and die off. Strips started to slough off. Our head nurse was horrified by what was happening. It looked like the dog was dying from the inside out. You could practically see the dead skin spread up the leg. We took blood samples, which showed there were massive degenerative changes to the liver as the toxins took effect. The liver enzymes were raised, indicating that the organ was struggling to neutralise the venom. This meant we had to be very careful what painkillers we used because certain analgesics can cause further damage to the liver. Thankfully the kidneys were stable, because once the kidneys are damaged, the change is irreversible.

She continued to deteriorate. Within forty-eight hours she began vomiting so we had to give her medicine to try and control that. Yet still she had a faint wag on her tail, and she used to look at us as if to say, 'I'm very poorly, but I'll be alright'. I could just tell she was determined to get better and that made me even more determined to help her through this.

But as the days progressed, her condition worsened. She stopped eating altogether so we boosted her energy via a glucose drip and syringed her with small quantities of a concentrated convalescent diet. More and more skin died and sloughed off. It spread over the entire leg and across her flanks and belly. The nurses were pulling handfuls of rotted flesh away. I'm not exaggerating when I say that over 25 per cent of the skin sloughed off that dog. With the skin off, the underlying musculature and bones were exposed. You could see her white, glistening ribs. She looked like one of the cadavers we used to practise on at Liverpool Veterinary School after an anatomy dissection.

After around five days our head nurse, Sarah, spoke to me.

'I think we need to consider putting her to sleep,' she said.

I had to agree that yes, euthanasia was an option, with the owner's consent, but that if we could just support the dog for a few more days, we would find the damage had peaked.

'She's not given up yet; I don't think we should,' I said. Sarah worked heroically and made it her personal challenge to save the patient.

The nurses were constantly bandaging the now skinless body with moisturised dressings to keep the tissues hydrated and it wasn't helping. Then I had an idea which I discussed with the nursing team, as this had become a massive team effort.

'Right,' I said, 'we're going to get a big bucket of udder cream and we're going to smear it all over this patient's body where the skin has sloughed off.'

They probably thought I'd taken leave of my senses, but I reckoned the gentle moisturising and mildly antiseptic cream would help fight infection and soothe the pain.

From then on, each day, our patient was slathered in the cream that was more commonly used for treating the udders of dairy cows, my thinking being that this was so gentle for the delicate tissue of our dairy friends that it would be equally gentle in this situation.

We did blood tests every day and the liver enzymes still rose, showing increasing damage. The liver is a very resilient organ and can regenerate but I was worried that the balance would tip and ultimately the liver would fail and our patient would die. The level of fortitude and grit this dog had shown was miraculous, but surely she couldn't continue fighting.

And then, after a week of touch-and-go, something remarkable happened. The enzyme level started to plateau out. The creeping skin necrosis stopped. Her breathing improved. She began to stabilise. A day later she started to eat a little bit on her own and her appetite continued to improve over the following days. I could see a little sparkle return to her dull eyes, and her wag, which never went away, got stronger. Life started to return to her. She was still in a terrible way but had turned a corner.

The following week was one of recovery. We continued with the udder cream and stopped the antibiotics, which didn't seem to be adding any further benefits. New skin started to grow, and after two weeks, we were able to send the dog home to her grateful owner.

As she was led out of the practice, wagging her tail vigorously, there wasn't a dry eye in the room. She went on to make a complete recovery, and when she came in some months later, the only evidence of the ordeal she'd been through were a few little scars where hair hadn't grown back on the new skin.

We were all amazed by the recovery. It was a true miracle.

'You know, all we do as veterinary surgeons sometimes is help nature,' I said to the head nurse. 'Nature is a wonderful thing. Sometimes it just needs a bit of a helping hand.'

Even now I know that others would have put her to sleep, and really, such decisions can be on a knife edge and can go either way. All you can do is make your best decision based on experience and the evidence in front of you. When I looked at the dog each morning and she looked at me with those doleful eyes and a bit of a wag of a tail, I knew she had a remarkable will to live.

Animals have a very different relationship with pain and discomfort than we do. They can put up with a lot. They're often stoic and rarely complain. And when things do go wrong, they tend to adapt as best they can and just get on with life. We can learn an awful lot from our four-legged patients.

A prime example of this was the case of Flynn the barn owl, who belonged to the Thirsk Bird of Prey Centre, where my nephew, who is a falconer, works. He's always had a love of animals and when he was at school, he used to cycle the six miles from Northallerton to the centre every week where he had a Saturday job, rain or shine. And that's the thing about birds of prey. You can't help falling in love with them. They're magnificent creatures, supremely adapted to do their job, keenly intelligent and – this might surprise some people – full of character. The centre has vultures, eagles, hawks, owls and many other species of birds, many of which take part in public displays, and each of them has their own personality. Flynn was one of their star performers and he was a lovely owl. He was very personable and loved people. The falconers at the centre all loved working with him. I have a saying that all animals and birds are special but some are more special than others. Flynn fell into the latter category.

All the birds at the centre are well looked after, and because they are always in close contact with the staff, any health problems are quickly spotted. Which is how one day it was noticed that one of Flynn's eyes was cloudy. The centre's manager, Kerry, called me out to have a look at him.

It was always a pleasure to take the trip out to the centre, which is a popular local attraction with around one hundred birds and fifty different species. In the tourist season it puts on several flying demonstrations each day with scores of birds flying around the centre and soaring over the beautiful Yorkshire countryside for the delight of visitors.

Kerry brought out Flynn and as expected, he was a model patient, sitting quietly and unperturbed while I had a good look at him. Unfortunately, it wasn't good news. Flynn had a lesion on his cornea, which told me he had a condition called corneal dystrophy. Sadly, this is not uncommon in animals and birds and is more often seen in older animals. Flynn was still a youngster. The worst part was that the condition is degenerative, progressive and often untreatable. Initially, I treated it as best I could with drops to try and slow the degeneration down but there was only ever one outcome, and sadly, the eye deteriorated and as such, became painful. The centre had a choice to make.

I spoke to Kerry.

'I'm afraid it's not going to get any better; it's going to become increasingly painful and he's going to start to struggle. We can remove his eye, or he could be put to sleep,' I explained.

Kerry was distraught at the thought of losing one of the best-loved members of the team. Indeed, they were all extremely attached to Flynn, and it turned out to be an easy choice to make. They didn't want Flynn to suffer and wanted to make the decision that was best for him.

Owls are wonderfully adaptable creatures and have such good hearing and such acute eyesight that they can perfectly adjust with one eye and modify their behaviour. It was decided that Flynn, who was bred in captivity and flew during the day, would lose his eye to save his life.

I added a note of caution.

'I have to warn you, Kerry,' I said, 'he may not survive the anaesthetic.'

'I understand, Peter,' she replied. 'Let's give it a go. He deserves a chance.'

The surgery was technical and tricky, and I never like removing eyes because, as a vet, it feels so barbaric. Owl's eyes are huge, and when I lifted this wet orb out of the socket and placed it on the stainless-steel tray by the side of the operating table, it looked up at me accusingly.

Nevertheless, Flynn survived the anaesthetic, and he went back to the centre where he recovered remarkably well thanks to the care he was afforded by the staff.

A few months later he was back doing what he loved and working with the team. He was the star turn when one of the visitors at the centre proposed to his girlfriend and had Flynn fly in with the engagement ring.

And that's the thing about animals. They don't have phobias and hang-ups about being able to cope. They either cope or they don't. We could all learn a thing or two from their attitude to life.

Flynn continued to work, and the staff watched him very closely because unfortunately, the kind of eye condition he had can be genetic and can affect both eyes. Sure enough, about nine months later I got a call I was dreading. It was Kerry again, who said she was worried about his other eye. I examined the little trooper again and our worst fears were confirmed. His remaining eye was starting to deteriorate. Again, I did what I could with medication, but the eye continued to deteriorate. It was becoming painful and he was going blind. His quality of life was declining, and, ultimately, we had to put him to sleep. It was a heart-breaking decision and everybody at the centre was in tears. I went there to perform this sad task so he didn't have the stress of travelling to the surgery. It was a very solemn occasion. They lost a valued member of the team. To tell the truth, I was upset as well. I had tears in my eyes putting him to sleep because he was such a fantastic, gutsy little character to have overcome adversity, but this was one battle he couldn't win.

I was reminded of Flynn a few years later when I met a little black cat called Lady who had been a stray and was taken in

Miracles can happen

by a bus company, where she earned her keep as a mouser. She was young but for inexplicable reasons she developed glaucoma in her right eye. It had come on suddenly and her eye was very swollen, around 50 per cent bigger than it should have been. Glaucoma is a very painful condition and the eye needed to be removed urgently.

Glaucoma is a serious condition because it causes fluid build-up in the eye. The pressure in the eye can build to such an extent that the internal structures are destroyed, rendering it useless.

Lady was a timid little thing, in a lot of pain, and so, with the help of one of the vet nurses, Hannah, I anaesthetised her so I could make a more detailed examination. It didn't take long to conclude that the eye's internal structures were already destroyed. Swollen and milky as it was, I shone my ophthalmoscope in and could see irretrievable damage. It was under so much pressure the eye wasn't far off rupturing and must have been causing her excruciating pain. It needed to come out as a matter of urgency.

Over the years I've taken many eyes out of cats and dogs, some of which the owners resented me doing at the time because they thought it made their pets look gruesome. But every single time I've done it, once the operation settled down, it was evident how much happier they were and so obvious how much pain they were living with, day in and day out.

With any eye removal there is a risk of haemorrhage, and the procedure looks particularly gruesome, but the risks outweigh the cruelty of allowing an animal to suffer by retaining a useless eye which in most cases is just a source of constant pain.

Lady's surgery went well and as I stitched her up, I wondered what her story was. How she'd ended up at the bus station. Cats are clever animals; they only go where they are welcome and they generally pick us, we don't pick them. If a cat doesn't like somewhere, they'll often go somewhere else where they feel more welcome.

'Cats aren't daft,' I told Hannah. 'Not like folks.'

Lady made a full recovery, and a few weeks later I went to Morse Coaches, based in a village just outside York, where Lady lived, to see how she was getting on. She was there, curled up in a box on a blanket on top of a printer in the office, happy as Larry. She lived there with Ginger, the firm's other mouser. The staff there admitted to me that although they were brought on board to be mousers and not pets, they had managed to ingratiate themselves with the staff there and generally led the life of Reilly, coming and going as they pleased from the administration office where two ladies worked away at the paperwork, often overseen by the cats. Sometimes they left their heated, cosy office and wandered around the yard to find a coach seat to sleep on. Having only one eye proved no impediment to Lady performing her day job and keeping the local vermin under control.

One of the other businesses in the area that we were often called out to help was Monk Park Farm near Bagby, which was a petting visitor attraction that had a menagerie of small and large animals, including alpacas, potbellied pigs, deer, llamas, wallabies and pigmy goats. One morning I received a call from the owner who explained that one of their wallabies had died. She was a mother and had been nursing her tiny albino joey, which was only a few days old. They found the poor mite sitting on top of the body of her mother, shivering, hungry and scared.

We had a dilemma. The joey, named Jilly, was not going to survive because with her mother dead, there was no way to feed her. The only option I had was to work out what milk substitute I could give her for her best chance of survival and for her to be hand-reared.

Most cases like this end in utter disaster. It's very time-consuming, you've got to get the correct consistency of the milk, correct intervals between feeds, as well as the correct volume and temperature.

Initially I chose a bitch milk replacer, which is a powdered milk with a balance of fats, sugars and proteins to mirror dog milk. I fed her first with a stomach tube to get her going and then started using a bottle. It worked, and Jilly drank hungrily. One of the girls who worked at Monk Park Farm, Sue, volunteered to be Jilly's carer. As it was a round-the-clock endeavour, Sue had to take Jilly home with her.

I was honest with her. 'Look,' I said, 'this may be a hiding to nothing.' Indeed, another similar case at Monk Park Farm didn't end so well. Maverick was a black alpaca baby whose mother died. He wouldn't feed and he was showing signs of pneumonia. He was only a few days old, and we had to stomach-tube him regularly. He had respiratory distress syndrome and he sadly didn't survive.

But Sue was determined to give it a go with Jilly, and off Jilly went with her new human mother.

Sue lived on a smallholding in a village just north of Thirsk and is a practical sort of lass. She was great with animals and not afraid of hard work. I've known Sue and her family for decades and knew she would put her heart and soul into Jilly's survival. I could see the determined look on her face when I told her the chances were slim. That look said: 'I'll show you.'

She took to Jilly and used a bottle to feed her every four hours, getting up in the middle of the night, looking after her with every fibre of her being. Jilly got stronger and stronger, and of course Sue became Jilly's mother. She hopped around the house after her as she did the housework, and as she got bigger, Sue used to take her out with her. They even went on days out to the seaside!

Eventually, Jilly got so big and strong that Sue knew it was time for her to go back and live with her wallaby mates at Monk Park Farm. Although she was domesticated, she fitted right back in, and whenever Sue was working, Jilly would hop over to say hello and they'd have a game of chase around the fields together.

It was a lovely success story and one that always makes me smile when I think about it. There's another case I look back on with fondness if I want to cheer myself up and it involves a family of farmers called the Bentleys. They own a farm in Bilsdale, one of the dales at the western edge of the North York Moors.

The farm had been in the Bentley family for several generations and was run by siblings Brian, Doreen and Cathy. They were old school and had grown up on the farm; it was in their blood. The place was meticulously run. They were people with common sense, not prone to dramatics. I remember our first conversation when I introduced myself as one of the new vets at Kirkgate.

'Good afternoon, I'm Peter. I've just started work with Alf and Donald at 23 Kirkgate.'

'Do you like lambings?'

'Yes, I do. I thoroughly enjoy the challenge.'

'Are you any good at 'em?'

'Well, I'll do my best.'

'Good. So, we know who to ring if we have a problem then, don't we?'

And that was it. Direct and to the point.

The irony about their concern for my lambing abilities was that the Bentleys were perfectly capable of lambing themselves and I cannot recall them ever getting into difficulties at lambing time and needing a vet. They knew their stock inside out. Over the years, I have got to know them well and developed a fondness for them.

Miracles can happen

They are salt-of-the-earth, lovely, genuine people. Sadly, there's only Brian and Doreen left now, and I still sometimes stop off and drop in some medication for them and we have a natter and put the world to rights. They're not silly and not really sentimental but have the sensible, common-sense approach that is a trait of lot of Yorkshire farmers. They were generous of spirit but had no airs or graces, and every Christmas they'd turn up with a bag of swedes at the surgery for Christmas lunches. Christmas was not the same without a Bentley swede.

They raised turkeys for Christmas and had cattle as well as sheep, which was why I had been called out to their farm one morning. One of their calves had taken ill. It had a very high temperature of 105 F and they called the practice asking for someone to see it urgently.

I arrived at the farm at 11am and there was nobody there, which was unusual, given the urgency of the request, but not a cause for concern as they had a lot of land and could have been in one of the fields attending to some other important matter. I went off to find the calf. It was in the calfhouse, and it was obvious which one it was. It was very poorly. Its lungs were going like bellows, breathing hot air into the morning chill, its nostrils flaring as it tried to take in sufficient oxygen. I knew by sight and the way it was behaving that it had bacterial pneumonia and needed significant treatment, quickly. For such conditions the required medication was antibiotics and anti-inflammatories, which I administered in a series of injections.

I could tell further how bad the poor thing was because as I injected it, it didn't move away, as most animals would, it just stood there and let me administer my treatments, with its head hung low, dejected and resigned to the intervention. I injected it intravenously to try and give it the best chance of survival, not a procedure our patients tolerated well as we used the jugular vein. Some people might say it intuitively knew I was trying to help. I did talk to it and try and soothe it. But the truth, however, was more likely that it had no strength left and couldn't be bothered to move away.

This is going to be touch-and-go, I thought to myself as I packed up my equipment. I fully expected a call later that day to tell me that the calf hadn't made it. I left and drove back to Thirsk with no confidence that my intervention had made any difference and got on with the rest of my day.

At 5pm I was given a message that had been called through from the Bentleys.

It read: 'Is vet coming because we'd like to stop him.'

I assumed the calf had died and called them back.

'Hello, Brian, it's Peter here—'

'We don't think you need to come now,' he interrupted.

'Oh dear, I'm sorry to hear that. I did try my best,' I explained.

Brian was perplexed.

'What do you mean?'

'I came this morning, no one was around, so I treated it. If I was a gambler, which I'm not, I would have given very low odds on it surviving. I tried but I thought then that it would be a miracle if it lived.'

Brian laughed.

'Well then, Peter, it's been a miracle. It's a lot better.'

I didn't know what to say. I was chuffed to bits. It was calls like that which make any vet feel as though they can walk on air.

I'm not exaggerating when I say some farmers, all they talk about are your failures. But from that day on, the Bentleys would always talk of that success. And fifteen years later they were still talking about it, whenever I dropped by.

Miracles can happen

'Tha' calf you treated, Peter, that were a miracle, weren't it? Do you remember?'

How could I ever forget? Certainly the Bentleys never will and I never tire of hearing about my success!

8

Strange cases

Winston the Labrador had a rather tragic start in life. One of a pair, his sibling was stillborn, so in his first months Winston missed the rough and tumble of having another puppy to play with, and perhaps that's why in later life he developed a strange habit.

Winston belonged to a good friend of mine, Mark, who is a former maths teacher, and his wife, Pam. They were both dog lovers. I play bridge with Mark each week and he is a very keen sportsman. He was a fantastic cricketer and was chair of the North Riding County Football Association. He is an upright character who loves life and lives it well.

Winston sometimes went to stay with Pam's parents, who were also dog fanatics. No one knows why Winston developed this strange habit, but it started one day when Winston was on one of his sleepovers. Pam's mother wore 'pop socks', which are the knee-high tights that older ladies sometimes wear. Winston was having a wander around the house, sniffing around as he did, and spied these pop socks laid out on a bed. For some reason, Winston

Strange cases

decided these items of hosiery would make a good meal and he devoured them. One can only imagine how tricky they would have been to swallow but Winston ate both so they must have been worth the effort.

Not long after, he started vomiting as his body tried to eject the foreign objects. When he didn't stop vomiting and was making no progress in ejecting the offending articles, he was taken to the Skeldale practice where I saw him. After a brief chat with Mark and Pam about his symptoms, it was apparent that one of the potential causes of his distress was that he'd eaten something that wasn't agreeing with him. To ascertain what was going on in his stomach, he was X-rayed. The problem with soft foreign bodies like pop socks is that they don't show up very well on radiographs. However, when I looked at the X-rays of Winston's abdomen, I could see a slight shadow and build-up of gas, which suggested there was something in there that didn't belong. Sometimes, when an animal eats something that can't be digested, it can be left to work its way through, but this only applies to small objects. The size of the shadow on the X-ray was big enough to give me reason to open him up, and so he was prepped for surgery.

It didn't take long to find out the cause once I had cut into his abdomen. Sure enough, there were the pop socks, which I teased out gently.

'Now, Winston,' I said to him as I worked, 'what do we have here?' There were two of them, bundled together and covered in digestive juices and bits of liquefied food. With raised eyebrows, I dropped them into a kidney bowl and set about stitching the patient back up.

After he'd come round, he stayed with us for observation. Generally, after such surgery an animal will stay for around twenty-four to forty-eight hours, until they've eaten and defecated. Two days later a sheepish Winston was sent away feeling sorry for himself, and I assumed that would be the last of the matter and that Winston had learned his lesson. However, it transpired that Winston obviously had developed a taste for footwear because three weeks later Pam was on the phone to the surgery.

'He's done it again,' she said, exasperated. 'This time it's socks.'

'Are you sure, Pam?' I asked.

'Absolutely sure, Peter,' she answered. 'I saw him. There was a pair of Mark's left on the bed and he jumped up quick as a flash and wolfed them down before I could get to him and pull them out of his mouth.'

I could only imagine Pam, who is quite athletic, making a dash to avert disaster and get the socks before Winston did, ending with a despairing dive onto the bed. But her efforts were in vain and now Winston was once more vomiting and in discomfort.

'You'd better bring him in again as a matter of urgency,' I advised.

Winston arrived soon after, his head hung low. He gave me a look as if to say, 'I've been a silly boy again, haven't I?'

'Oh, Winston,' I said. 'What have you done?'

We didn't need to X-ray him this time as we had an eyewitness, and sure enough, when he was opened again on the operating table, there in his stomach were a pair of dark men's cotton socks.

Once again, Winston was stitched up and sent away looking sorry for himself after he'd recovered.

From that day on, things changed in Mark and Pam's house. Winston needed to be weaned off his strange addiction and so hosiery, socks and other undergarments were kept under lock and key, out of temptation's way. Winston went cold turkey, and it appeared to work until some years later when Mark and his sons, who were decent cricketers like their father, went to a cricket match near Wetherby and took Winston along with them. The local team were playing a team visiting from Australia and the Aussies had batted. It was a warm day and some of the players had left their pads out in the sun and placed their sweaty socks on top of them to dry. Winston was having a wander around when he spied these abandoned morsels and couldn't help himself. He bounded over to the pads, which would have looked and smelled like a sock buffet to him, and before anyone could do anything, Winston had gulped down a sock.

For the third time, Winston found himself back at Skeldale as an urgent admission, on the operating table, abdomen open with me standing over him, fishing out a sock. The operation was another success, but when Winston left us this time I did crouch down and explain to him that enough was enough and it was time to stop.

The funny postscript to the story is what happened to that last sock after it was removed from Winston's gut. Winston's notoriety spread to Australia and the visiting team thought the sock, which was returned to its owner, had great merit as a trophy. And so there is now an annual match on the other side of the world in which teams play for Winston's trophy.

Heaven knows why animals do it, but bye 'eck they eat some strange things. I've pulled all manner of strange foreign objects out of stomachs.

There was the case of Khufu the cat who belonged to the wife of one of our farming clients at Skeldale. Trish was a very caring lady who really nurtured her animals and looked after them extremely well. She would always have something ready to eat if I was paying a visit to her husband on the farm. Being a farmer, Trish used to get herself involved with the animals if any of them were ill, especially if nursing was involved, where she really excelled. She had horses at the farm and as soon as something was wrong with one of them, she would be on the phone asking for a vet to visit, which we were only too pleased to do because she was a prolific baker and there was always something tasty on offer after we'd conducted whatever examination and treatments were required. She had two Siamese cats, one of which was Khufu, and they were free to roam the house. If anything was wrong with one of them, she'd bring them in to the practice right away. She wasn't the kind of person who would wait to see how things go before taking action.

One day she came in with Khufu and explained that he was having difficulty eating. Whatever was troubling him didn't seem to be affecting him when I got him out of his carrier and he hopped off the surface and had a good wander round the examination room, taking in all the new and unusual smells.

I started to examine him. I listened to his chest, which sounded fine, and looked in his mouth to see if he had any problems with his teeth, gums or throat. Everything looked okay. I palpated his abdomen and noticed something unusual.

A cat's stomach is located mainly under the ribcage, and by gently pressing just behind the last rib I could feel something solid. I frowned. It felt as if it could be some sort of hard tumour.

Oh no, I thought to myself, *this may well be something extremely serious, and sadly at such a young age may be the end for Khufu.*

In veterinary practice we are encouraged to gather as much evidence as possible, which in some cases can mean lots of expensive scans and tests, and before I gave any devastating news to Khufu's owners, I needed to be sure. But I also didn't want to be overly optimistic in case my fears were confirmed. Honesty is always the best policy.

Strange cases

'There is something in his stomach,' I explained. 'It could be any number of things, so I'll do some tests to try and get a clearer picture of what we're dealing with.'

I took some blood from him, and we ran tests, but the results showed nothing of any significance. So then we X-rayed him. The resulting image was baffling. Inside his stomach there was a bizarrely-shaped circular mass. I'd never seen anything quite like it, but it looked ominous.

I explained to his owner that I would need to operate and that although I wasn't sure, she should prepare herself for bad news.

'Because there's something strange going on inside him,' I said. 'It could be a nasty tumour. The X-rays are quite confusing.'

Khufu was admitted for surgery and Rachel, our hardworking head nurse, assisted me, as she often did with difficult surgeries.

I opened his abdomen and got to his stomach, which was distended beyond belief and quite knobbly.

This is not going to end well, I thought as I cut into it, expecting to find some kind of grotesque, knobbly, cancerous mass.

Instead, as the stomach lining parted, I stopped and blinked.

'What's that?' I asked.

I reached in carefully and pulled out an elasticated fabric ring. I held it up to get a better look.

Rachel, who was standing next to me, started to laugh.

'It's a hairband,' she said, having worn many herself. I freely admit here I had no use for such accessories in my wardrobe.

'A hairband!' I exclaimed. 'What's he doing eating hairbands?'

And it was clear on further probing there were plenty more left inside him.

Rachel went to get a kidney bowl, and one after another I lifted these things out of Khufu's stomach. We started counting.

'One, two, three—'

Some of them had long hair wrapped around them.

'—seven, eight, nine—'

It kept going. It was like one of those magic tricks where the magician pulls a never-ending handkerchief from his pocket.

There were thirteen in total. How they all fitted into this cat's stomach I'll never know. When I finished and they were piled up in the kidney bowl, I could scarcely believe what I was looking at. I kept looking at the kidney bowl and then looking at Khufu on the table.

What goes on in your head, boy? I thought to myself.

Once Khufu had been stitched up and had recovered, he was returned to his owner, along with the hairband collection.

'I thought I was running a bit short of them,' she said.

I pondered the great mystery of why a cat would get such a taste for hairbands that he would almost kill himself gorging on them and the only answer that made sense was that Khufu associated them with his owner, whom he obviously adored. Cats have a keen sense of smell, and these bands would have his owner's scent on them. Perhaps he got comfort by chewing on them. Perhaps that too was the reason Winston started on his sock diet. Maybe they reminded him of his owners, or people he loved, and he got a taste for them. Maybe the pop socks were a gateway that led him to crave more substantial footwear. Who knows where it might end? Wellington boots?

More recently I was left pondering these things again when I removed a piece of leathery material from a cocker spaniel's stomach that appeared to have a plastic nipple attached to it. I was puzzled as to what it was before a colleague flipped it over and showed me that it was part of a football. What I thought was a nipple was the valve. Was this a budding footballer who had got totally carried away with the sport? Who knows?

Strange cases

Why would a dog eat that? I wondered.

Less puzzling was the case of Wesley, the border terrier who was rushed into Skeldale having consumed an oven glove. His owner also had a snake named Snakey. She called the surgery one day in a real flap.

'Wesley's eaten me oven glove,' she said, panicking.

'You'd better bring him in,' I advised.

She came in, Wesley came in, and the remaining remnants of the glove came in.

'Look. He's eaten half of it,' she said, gesturing at the ragged, fat-soaked piece of material she'd placed on the examination table.

'Are you sure he's swallowed it?' I asked, in the vain hope that perhaps Wesley had thought he'd grabbed a nice pork chop but then realised it was far too tough to eat and left it.

'Definitely,' she asserted. 'I looked everywhere and half of it has gone.'

I looked down at Wesley who was looking at me, wagging his tail, bright as a button. He certainly wasn't in any pain or discomfort. Indeed, dare I say it, he was looking rather pleased with himself.

'How is he in himself?' I asked.

'He's been sick a couple of times, but nothing came up. I know he's definitely eaten it,' she reasserted.

I leaned down to have a proper look at him and a feel around his tummy, which he seemed to enjoy. Nothing was evident on clinical examination, but an oven glove would be difficult to feel, soaked and softened by digestive juices in Wesley's stomach.

'We'll have to X-ray him,' I explained.

Sure enough, the X-ray showed an air pocket, and a vague outline of semi-radio-opaque material, which is one of the indicators of soft foreign bodies in a digestive tract. Judging by the remains of the glove, Wesley had made a good job of ingesting as much as he could and there was a significant amount inside him. It was robust material and looked as if it was unlikely to pass through him on its own, so the only option was to remove it surgically, which I did, and thankfully Wesley made a full recovery. Unlike the socks and hairbands, it was obvious why Wesley had tried to snaffle the oven glove, which would have smelled of cooked meat and been covered in dried fat and juices.

Wesley had come undone in his search for tasty morsels, which is often a route to misfortune. Another case involved a Skeldale client called Tony Woodcock, who was an area manager for a large poultry company in the area. He came by one Sunday morning with his border terrier, and had been out fishing on the Cod Beck, the stream that runs through Thirsk.

Tony had put down a hook momentarily which was baited with some chopped pork and the dog had gobbled it down quickly, unable to resist such a temptation.

Again, I used X-rays to locate the offending item and found that it was trapped in the gullet over the top of the heart. I couldn't go down through the tissue with grabbers to pull it back because the barb would have hooked into the gullet and possibly through to the heart. One option was a thoracotomy, which involves opening the chest to get to the chest cavity and the gullet, but this is a risky operation in veterinary practice. The other option was to use something to try to push the hook down into the stomach, from where it could be retrieved via a much easier surgical technique.

When our luncheon-meat-loving patient was anaesthetised, I used an endoscope to examine the hook. It was clear it had not punctured the gullet lining and therefore I could safely try and manoeuvre it down.

Strange cases

Veterinary surgery is often about improvising, and, in that case, I used a length of plastic tubing to gently nudge the hook further along the digestive system where I successfully removed it in the same way I dealt with Wesley and the other reprobates who had eaten things they shouldn't have.

In all these cases, a knowledge of the intestinal diameter as well as the size and shape of the foreign body within the patient, and a common-sense approach, are needed to work out whether something is going to be passed naturally through the rectum or whether it's going to cause damage, like the fishing hook, or whether it's too big to pass naturally and needs to be removed surgically.

Sewing needles are another common object that animals seem to swallow, often with thread attached. I have no idea why; it always perplexes me. The thing about sewing needles is that they often stick on the way into the alimentary canal, in the throat, or on the way out, at the anus, in which case you're presented with a dog with a bit of sewing thread hanging out of their bottom. In those cases, you can often remove the offending article using rectally inserted forceps. That a needle can pass all the way through a dog or cat and emerge from the other end just shows how robust and wonderful the alimentary system is. It may not be easy for a camel to pass through the eye of a needle, as it says in the Bible, but in some cases it's relatively easy for a needle to go through the alimentary tract of a dog.

Some animals very quickly develop vices, like a ten-week-old Rottweiler puppy I recently saw that developed a taste for pebbles. He came in with his owner, who was only a young chap himself. He'd wanted a dog for years and his parents granted his wish when they felt he was responsible enough to look after one. He took his pet-owning responsibilities very seriously and bought books to learn as much about looking after dogs as possible. He came to the practice to get the pup vaccinated, and less than a couple of weeks later he returned in a very concerned state because he'd been out in the garden getting his puppy used to his lead, when as quick as a flash the pup grabbed some pebbles and swallowed them before he had a chance to react.

Why, I asked myself, would an animal want to eat pebbles? They have no flavour, they would be hard, and it didn't even sound like it had been playing with one and swallowed it accidentally. On chatting to the distraught owner, it seemed the puppy was hell-bent on swallowing as many as possible.

The young owner had worry etched over his face.

'Me dog's ate some stones; what'll happen?' he asked.

I asked what size the stones were, and he explained, using his fingers and thumb, that they were quite substantial. As we were obviously dealing with a young puppy, it only had puppy-sized intestines, and so we X-rayed him to be sure, and the image showed these stones clearly sitting in the stomach and that they would have been unlikely to pass through the narrow small intestine on their own. We had to surgically remove them. The poor lad who owned him was beating himself up and blaming himself.

I told him not to be so hard on himself because sometimes dogs will just eat something for no obvious reason to us.

'It will never happen again,' the young man promised. I knew he meant it by the determined look on his face.

The pebbles were dutifully removed, and I chewed over in my head, why would this puppy want to eat such things?

Later in the day whilst the puppy was recovering from the operation, one of the nurses took him out to the car park so he could get some fresh air and hopefully pass urine and, more relevantly, faeces.

Strange cases

It was his first trip outside since the surgery and he stepped outdoors confidently and sniffed the air. He was on a lead and started pulling, his tail wagging. He seemed to be focussed on something that he was heading towards. The nurse allowed him to go where he wanted but it soon became apparent he was hatching a plan. He pulled her to a patch of gravel and, lo and behold, he bent down instantly and grabbed a pebble to eat. The nurse immediately opened his mouth and removed it from his clamped jaws before he could swallow. It was obvious that the antics that had brought him to the surgery were clearly premeditated and not a one-off. This puppy had a dangerous penchant for pebbles and his owner was going to have to be extremely careful. When he came to collect him we warned him that from then on they should keep him away from pebbles and stones and keep a close eye on him when he was out. Hopefully he grew out of his odd craving as we did not see him again.

But the most bizarre thing I ever retrieved from inside an animal was back in the Kirkgate years when the owner of a local garage brought his Labrador in because she was being sick. I thought she had picked up some sort of bug, but I checked her and could feel something solid in her duodenum, the first part of the small intestine. When she was X-rayed, the problem was as clear as day. The dog had swallowed a spark plug (a car's engine part, tubular and about three inches long). There it was, plain to see, as clear as day. How she had even managed to swallow it, or why, was beyond me. Maybe it had something to do with hero worship? Maybe she'd watched her beloved owner handle these items on many occasions and associated them with him?

It's not just strange objects that can cause animals problems when eaten. Sometimes too much food, or the wrong type of food can have problematic consequences too, which are sometimes even fatal. Cattle can suffer from a condition called barley poisoning, for example. This occurs occasionally when they're fed on barley to fatten them. If this is introduced too quickly and they gorge on it, the barley ferments away in their stomach and produces methane and other gases. Adult cattle have four stomachs, the largest of which is called the rumen and it's like a huge fermenting vat. If the barley ferments too quickly it produces a lot of gas which has to be released by either passing down, so to speak, or up through a very efficient belching process. If they can't expel the fermentation gas quickly enough, it builds up in the rumen, grossly distending it. This can then put massive pressure on other organs and major blood vessels, resulting in circulatory shock and sudden death. If the gas build-up is less severe, these cattle can become drunk and are often found staggering about in a disorientated fashion. This less acute form of barley poisoning often results in diarrhoea and severe dehydration. This toxic effect can also be fatal.

Dogs regularly end up in trouble after eating food they shouldn't, like Stonker and Sausage, two terriers who were rushed in one night after gorging on a packet of raisins they'd found. Raisins can be toxic in dogs, so I saw them straight away. I was told that they'd eaten half a pound of the dried fruit each. In the old days we would give such cases washing soda crystals to induce vomiting, and we'd always have a box in Kirkgate for such eventualities, but this is hard to come by in this day and age. A chunk of it down the dog's throat would soon have them honking and heaving away. Nowadays we use apomorphine, which is a very strong emetic, meaning it induces pronounced vomiting. A small quantity administered intramuscularly will encourage a dog to vomit up to a dozen times. I used it on both Sausage and Stonker, and they regurgitated huge quantities of raisins all over the consulting room floor. This

Strange cases

emergency was filmed for *The Yorkshire Vet*, and the story ended with them happily trotting off home with no ill effects from their dried fruit feast. What the film crew failed to capture was me on my hands and knees just before midnight cleaning the copious piles of vomit from the consulting room floor. Such is the glamorous life of a vet!

One of the strangest cases of a foreign body in an animal did not even involve eating. The patient was a horse called McCoy who belonged to a lady called Debbie who was well-versed and highly experienced in the equine world. She took part in various equine competitions and competed at a high level. McCoy was one of her favourite and best geldings and he had a swelling on his jawline that was discharging pus. Despite Debbie's best efforts, the wound wouldn't heal.

When I read the entry in the practice day book to visit McCoy I thought, *This'll be an easy job.* I drove to the stables full of blind confidence, assuming that a good clean-up with antiseptic and a course of antibiotics would sort out the problem in no time.

Sure enough, when I examined the good-natured patient, my initial prognosis was confirmed. The wound was not severe but there was swelling and tenderness over the jaw and an infection which was causing a discharge on the underside of the jawbone. I cleaned the wound up, applied antiseptic and gave a shot of good old-fashioned penicillin and thought that would do the trick. Over the following days it improved but did not heal completely. It did seem to be a little more stubborn than I was expecting.

I revisited McCoy and gave him a longer course of antibiotics to help settle it down.

'That should sort it out,' I told Debbie.

I heard nothing and assumed it had healed, but a few weeks later Debbie was back on the phone.

'The discharge has increased again,' she explained. 'I'm getting a lot more out now. Would you come out and have another look at him, please?'

I went back and was baffled. There was no glandular enlargement. There was no other swelling, but she was right, the discharge, having seemingly improved on the antibiotics, had worsened again. I decided to give McCoy a week's course of injectable antibiotics and returned daily to inject him, which was no problem because he was a good patient and didn't mind being jabbed. Again, he improved, but after a week or so, the discharging wound deteriorated and started oozing pus yet again.

This pattern which had developed was beginning to look like what we call a foreign body reaction. Could McCoy have got a thorn or some other piece of debris lodged in his subcutaneous tissues? Finding foreign bodies which are causing discharging tracts from the body can be incredibly difficult to locate in animals. It can literally be like looking for a needle in a haystack.

It was clear that whatever was causing McCoy's problem was not going to clear up on its own, so when I returned, I sedated him to keep him calm in order to investigate the wound and find the source of the problem.

He was such a good patient and stood still as I started my work. I found the tract through which the pus was draining and started to dissect along it deeper and deeper into the tissues and musculature on the inner side of McCoy's jawbone. I had to be careful because, remembering my anatomy classes, I knew the area carried several significant blood vessels. I enlarged the tract and followed it down until I could get my whole finger inside this cavernous tract on the inside of the mandible. When the full length of my finger was in the tract, I felt something right at the end of my fingertip. It was hard and sharp.

Strange cases

What on earth is that? I thought to myself.

The owner was watching intently as I stood there frowning, with my finger deep in the underside of her prize gelding's jaw.

'There's something in here that shouldn't be,' I told her. 'I haven't a clue what it is.'

I formulated a plan. I had crocodile forceps, which have scissor-like handles attached to a long, thin stem with a grabber on the end. I thought that if I could get the forceps into the hole and guide them along the side of my finger, I could reach the object and try to pull it out. It was a tricky operation and I was concerned that I might clip a blood vessel. With my finger still inside the hole, I used my free hand to operate the forceps and tried to get a grip on whatever it was inside McCoy's jaw. I pulled them back and out of the hole. Nothing. The grip must have slipped. I went in again, grabbed and pulled. Again, nothing. I went in a third time, felt the forceps grate against and grip the object and gave them a wobble. I carefully pulled and felt a bit of give. When I pulled the gripper free from the discharging hole, there was something white, curved and bloody clasped in them.

'What the bloody hell is that?' I said, holding it up to get a closer look.

It was a tooth.

'Unbelievable!' I exclaimed. 'It would seem McCoy has had his head in a hedgeback and startled either a rat, a weasel or a stoat and been bitten. The perpetrator's tooth has obviously been wrenched out as McCoy pulled his head back abruptly and lodged under the skin on the inside of his jawbone'

Debbie explained that one of McCoy's favourite pastimes was poking his head into the hedgeback in his field, which confirmed my theory.

It had seemed such a simple little job on my first visit to see McCoy.

There's no accounting for why animals stick their heads in the places they do. I suppose curiosity gets the better of them. McCoy has hopefully learned his lesson, but others are more stubborn, such as Joe the pygmy goat who lived at Monk Park Farm and developed a habit that drove his owners to distraction.

'I'm bloody sick of this goat,' was how the conversation started when I was called out to deal with Joe.

He was a very angelic-looking creature with horns that raked back over the rear of the head.

The cause of consternation was his habit of sticking his head through the wire mesh of the fence that enclosed the field in which he lived. For many animals, the grass is always greener on the other side of their enclosures and Joe was no exception. He could squeeze his head through the fence but then found it impossible to withdraw it due to his magnificent horns. The staff at the farm were having to release Joe up to eight times a day.

And that wasn't the worst of it. Joe had been teaching the other goats his newly learned trick as well. Sometimes visitors would be greeted by the sight of four or five goats with their heads sticking through the fencing, unable to get free.

'Please can you dehorn him for me, Peter, before they all start doing it?' said Joe's owner. 'I'm bloody sick of this now!'

Well, goats are tricky to dehorn. They have sizeable blood vessels in their horns as they get older and removing them can result in serious haemorrhage. Also, the local anaesthetic used for cows is toxic in goats, so they have to be given a general anaesthetic in order to carry out the procedure. None of this is without risk.

Joe was taken to Skeldale in a trailer, and we put him on the operating table, put a mask over his face and turned on the gaseous anaesthetic until he drifted off to sleep. His horns were taken off

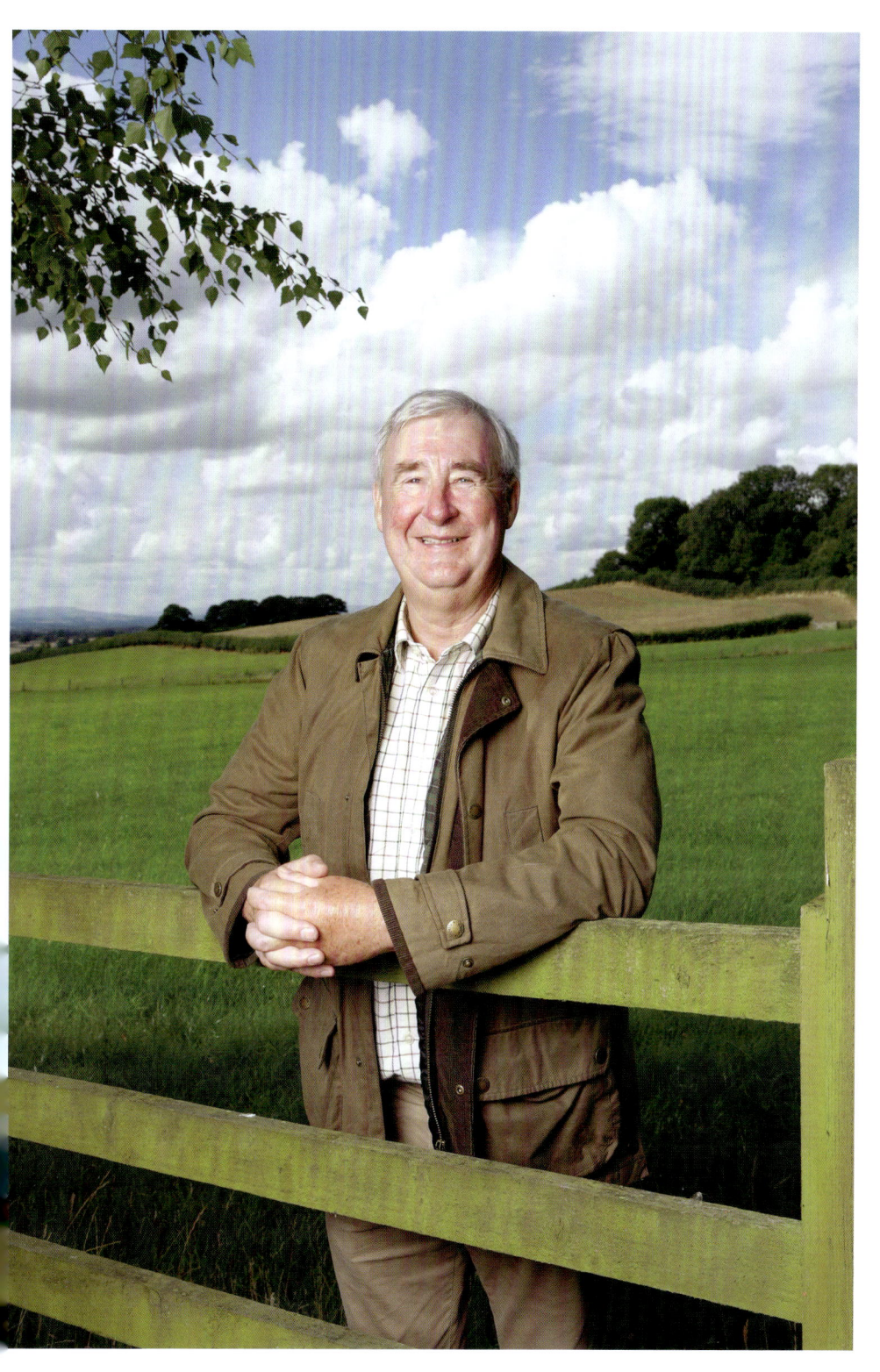

At home – a happy place to be.
Photograph: Barry Marsden Photography

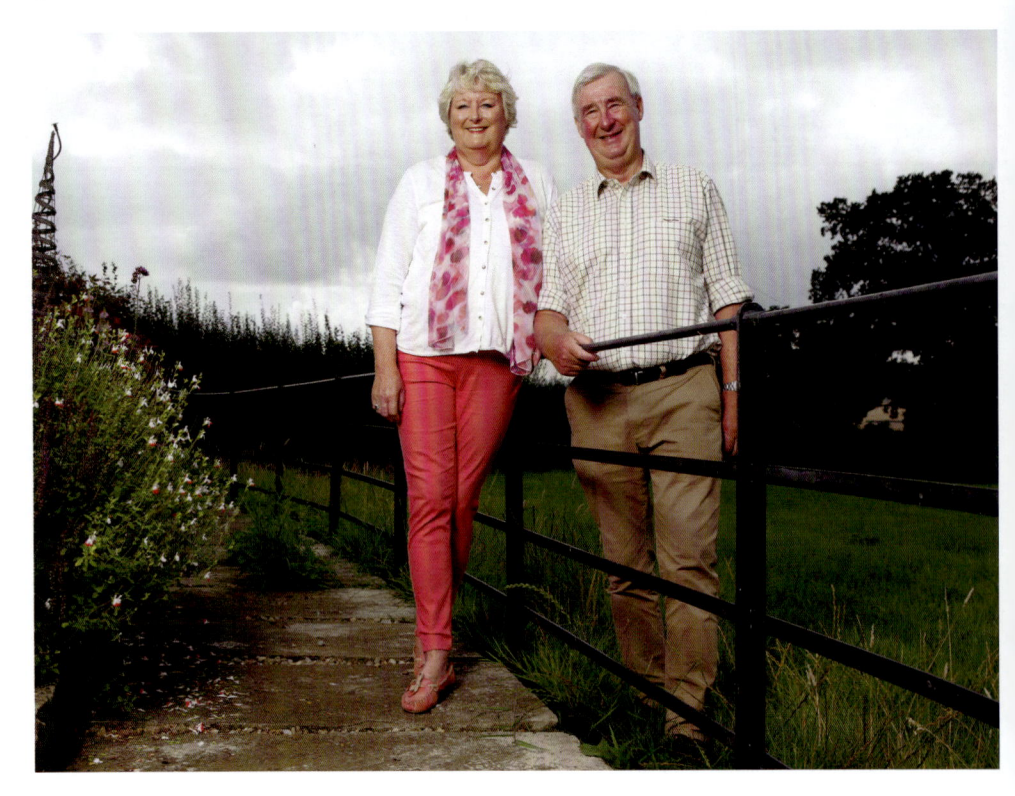

Me with the long-suffering Lin in the garden at home.
Photograph: Barry Marsden Photography

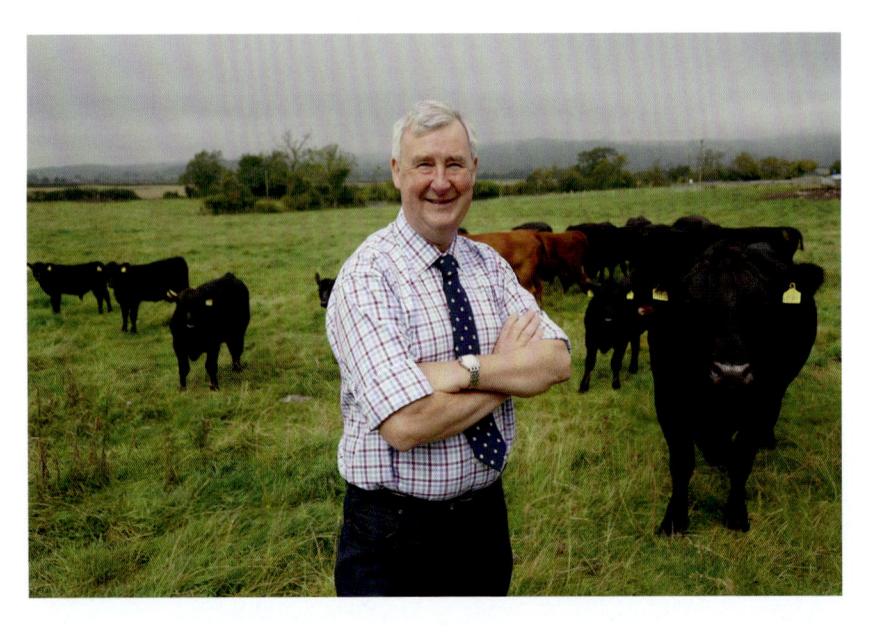

I am always happy when amongst a herd of cattle.
Photograph: Courtesy of Daisybeck Studios/Motion Content Group

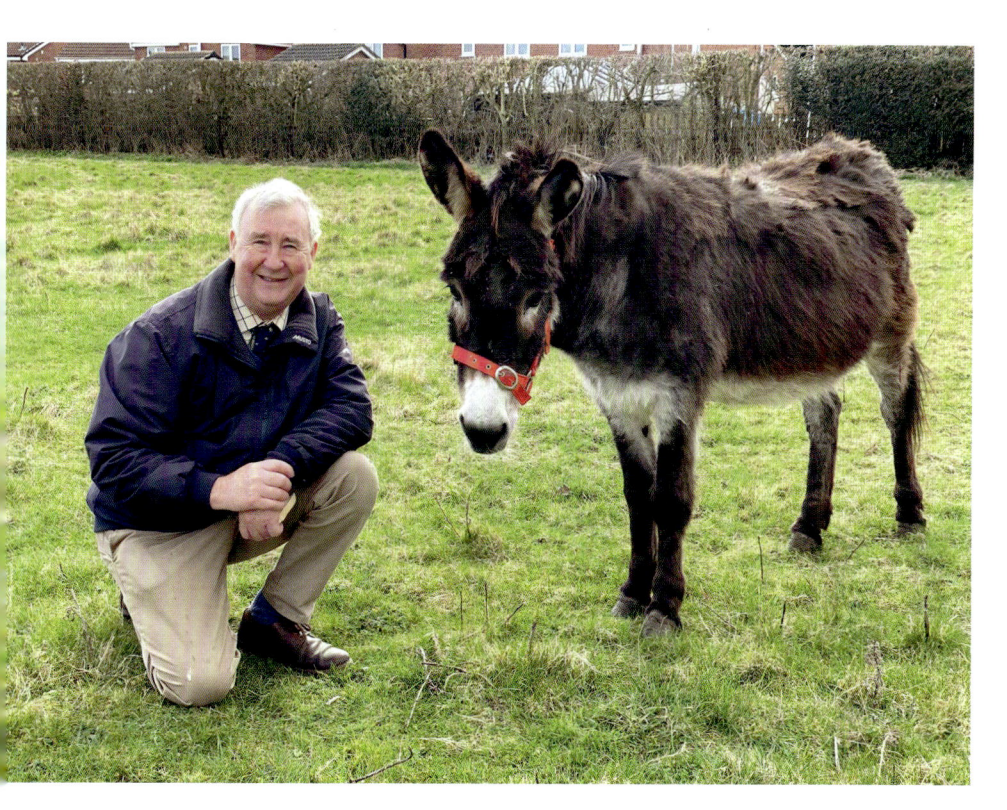

Posing with Steve and Jean Green's donkey Sybil, who was rather sad after losing her companion Mabel.
Photograph: Courtesy of Daisybeck Studios/Motion Content Group

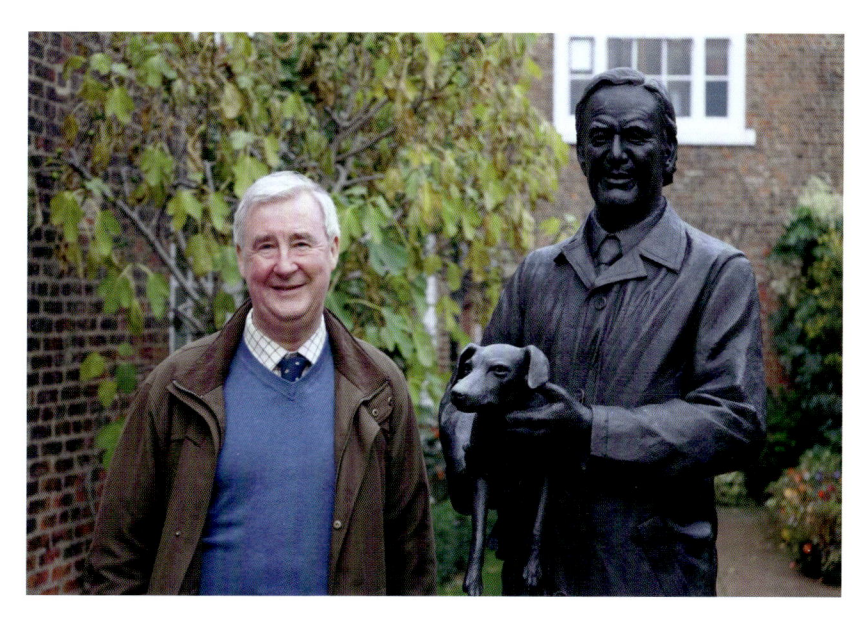

With the statue of Alf Wight in the garden of the old Kirkgate surgery, which is now *The World of James Herriot* tourist attraction.
Photograph: Author's own

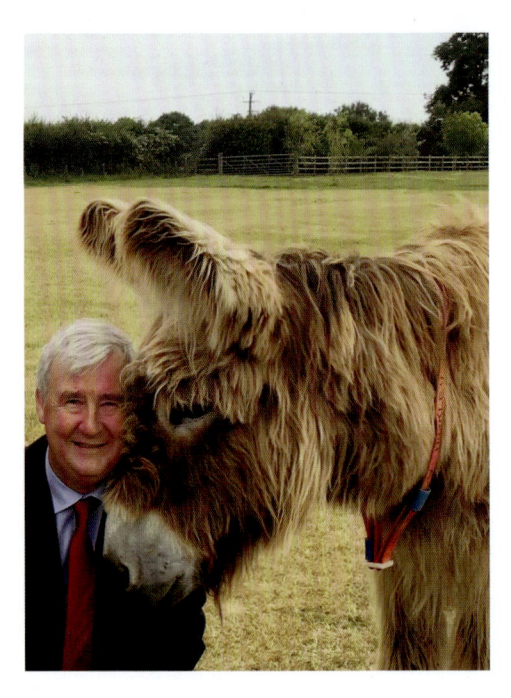

Making a new friend. A beautiful Poitou donkey at The Donkey Sanctuary in Devon.
Photograph: Author's own

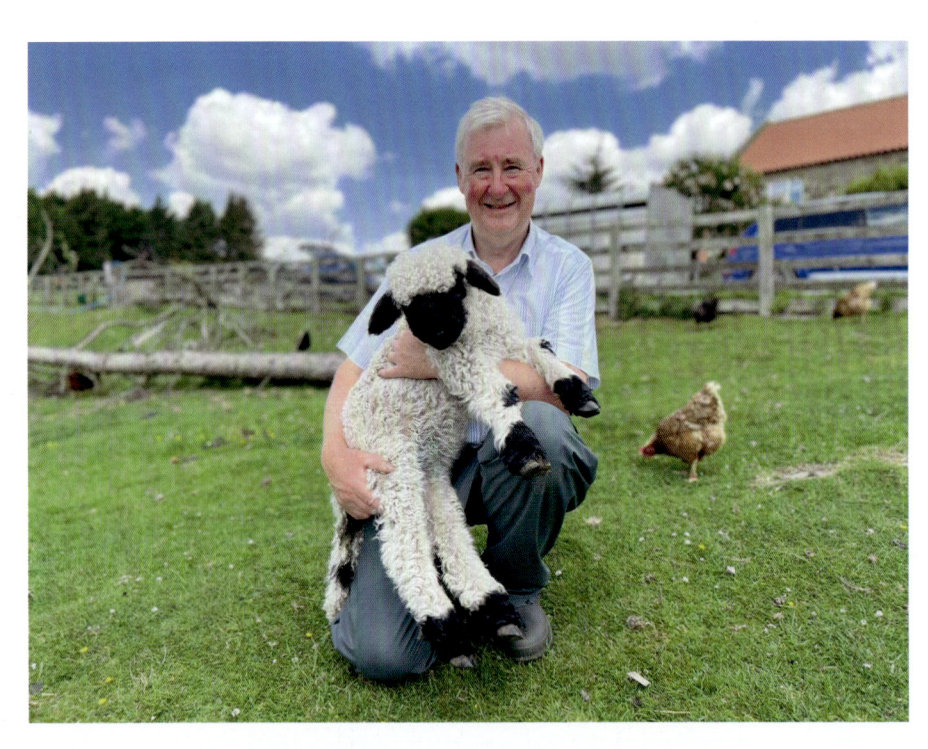

Having a cuddle with a striking Valais Blacknose lamb.
Photograph: Courtesy of Daisybeck Studios/Motion Content Group

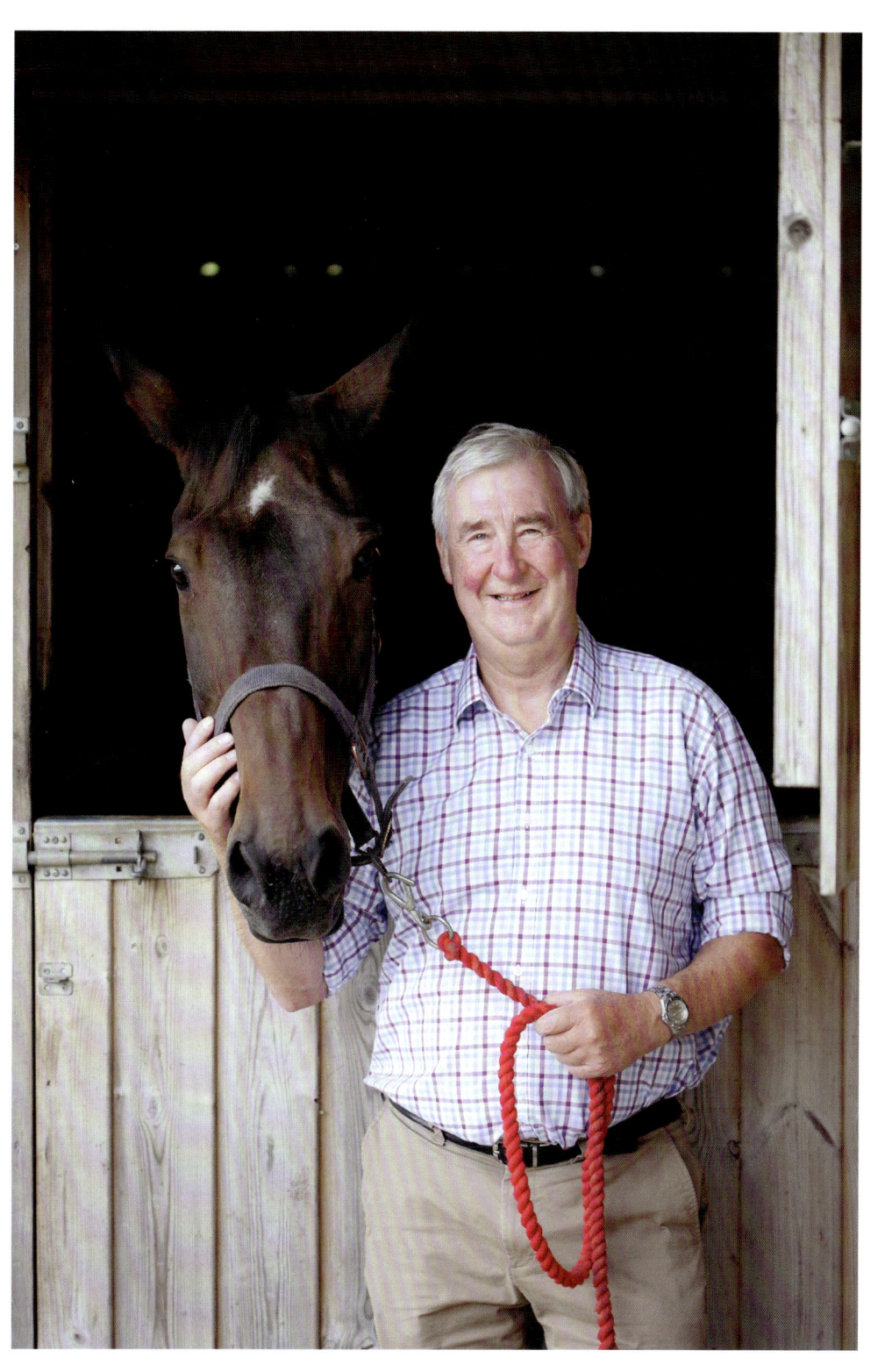

Dylan, our much-loved neighbour's horse.
Photograph: Barry Marsden Photography

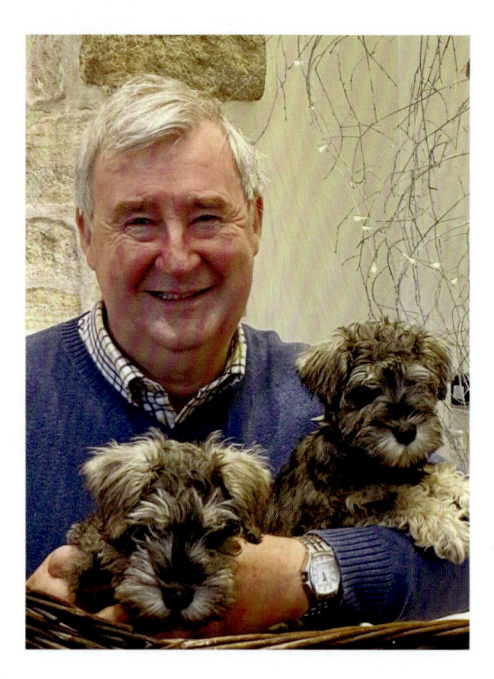

Two beautiful Schnauzer puppies. You can see the mischief on their faces.
Photograph: Author's own

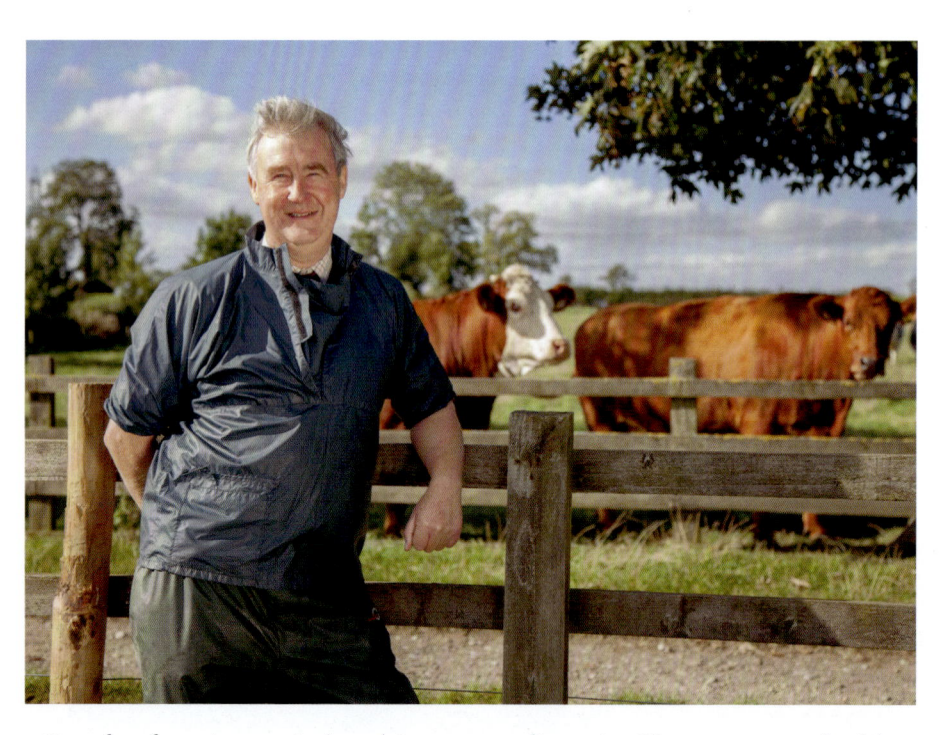

One of my favourite morning's work is pregnancy diagnosing. You can see a couple of the ladies in the background.
Photograph: Courtesy of Daisybeck Studios/Motion Content Group

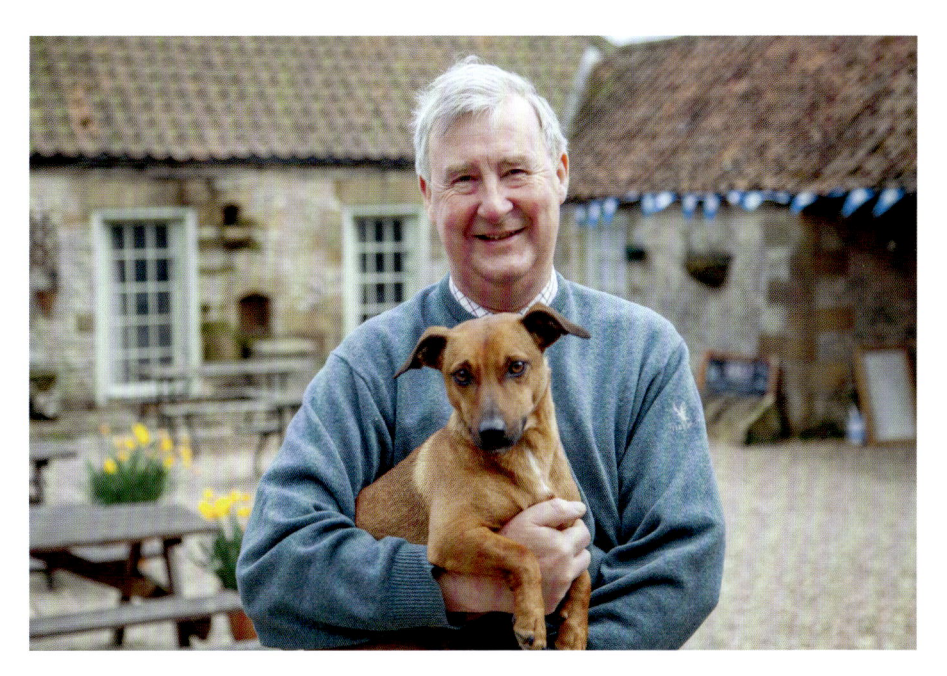

Here is Stonker who lives in a tearoom. He stole and ate a whole packet of raisins, which are poisonous to dogs, so he had to pay me an urgent visit.

Photograph: Courtesy of Daisybeck Studios/Motion Content Group

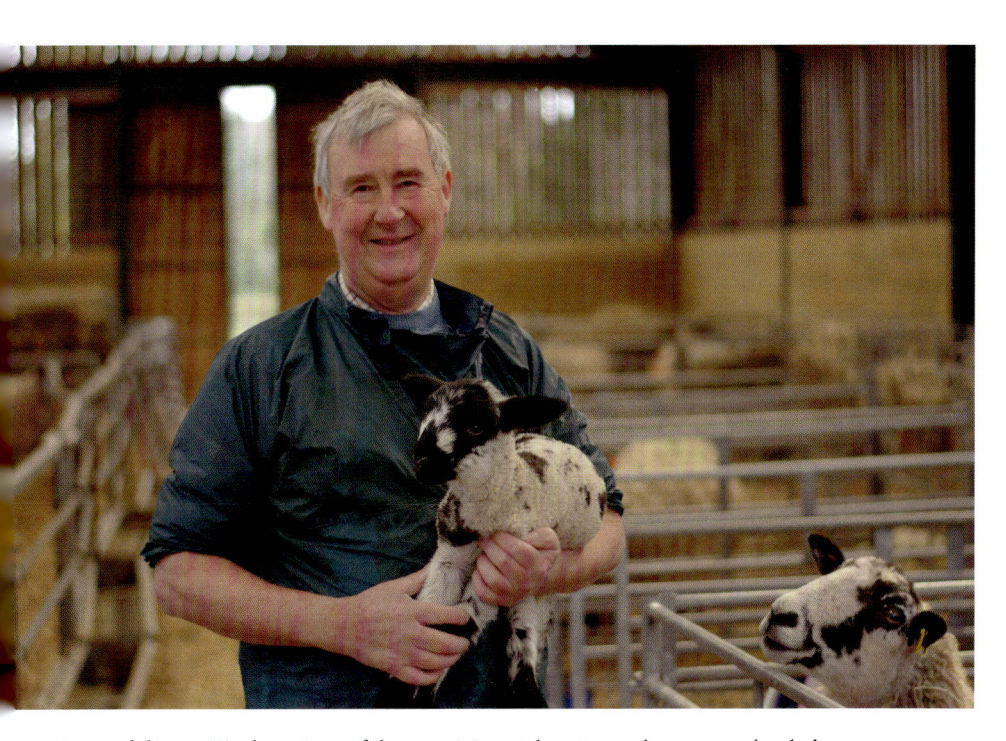

A new delivery. The best time of the year. Mum is keeping a close eye on her baby to ensure she comes to no harm.

Photograph: Courtesy of Daisybeck Studios/Motion Content Group

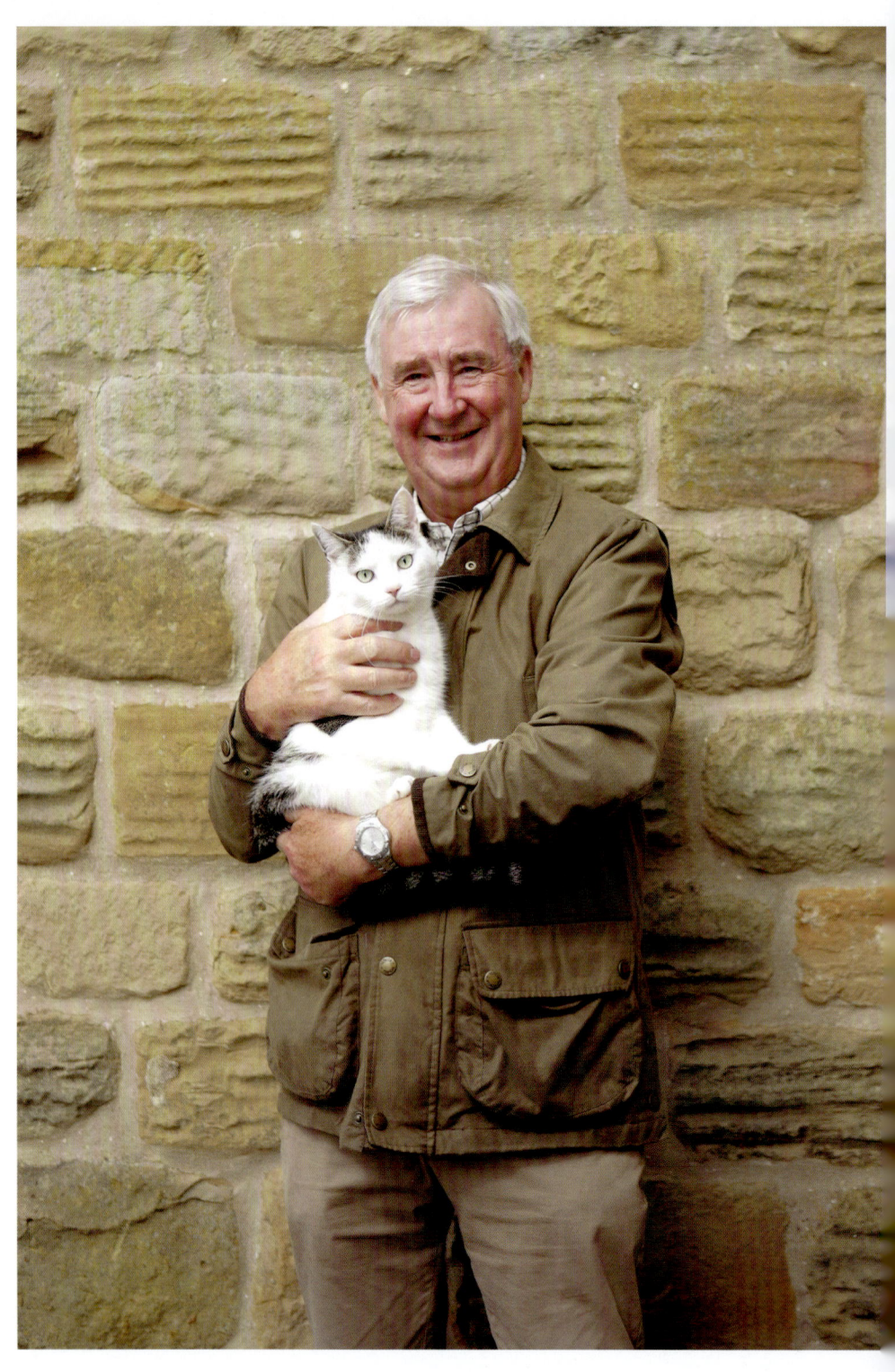

A rare picture of Toddy our rescued cat. He is usually far too superior and aloof to be photographed. You can see the look of disgust on his face!
Photograph: Barry Marsden Photography

with a cheese-wire type cutting device and a hacksaw and then I used a hot disbudding iron to cauterise them and stop them growing back.

The operation went without a hitch and when Joe returned minus his horns he could no longer wedge himself in the fence, and he stopped his strange behaviour when he realised he could no longer play the game with his carers, in which they arrived several times a day to release him. Without their ringleader the other goats also stopped sticking their heads through the fence as well.

Seemingly, the grass was no longer greener on the other side.

9

Cock and bull stories

They call me 'The Testicle King of Thirsk'. My prowess at depriving animals of their gonads is frequently highlighted on the small screen during episodes of *The Yorkshire Vet*, but truth be told, my castrating career stretches way back to the Kirkgate years when Alf Wight would explain that removing the testicles technically wasn't a difficult procedure, but the hard part was persuading your patient he didn't need them anymore. For farm animals, where we haven't the luxury of an operating theatre and time, there are different methods used for castration. When an animal is very young, you can use a special elasticated band which encloses the base of the scrotum and pinches off the blood supply to the testicles. Within a week or so the testicles wither and drop off, like unpicked plums. The method I was brought up with, and use most frequently, is the bloodless method carried out using an apparatus called a Burdizzo. These are heavy steel pliers with a long tapered head that pinch and crush the spermatic cord and blood vessels to the testicles (it's at this point male readers will be crossing their legs). The procedure takes seconds, and a local anaesthetic

Cock and bull stories

is used to numb the site. After the procedure, the testicles wither over a period of time and die off. Burdizzos come in two sizes: smaller ones for goats and sheep and larger ones for bulls. The other option is to use a local anaesthetic, make a large incision through the scrotum, pull out the testicle and then either tie the blood vessels off or pull and twist, the recoil of which causes the blood vessels to constrict. There is a reasonable likelihood in these cases that some animals might bleed, especially larger ones, and I've known one or two to bleed to death. There is also a greater risk of infection in summer due to flies pestering the wound site. Some vets in other practices would always insist on cutting, but at Kirkgate we favoured the Burdizzo method.

Bull castrations are hard work, and in my younger days I'd be sent out to these 'rodeos' in trepidation of being kicked black and blue by any number of bulls that didn't want to be deprived of their reproductive equipment. As a rule of thumb, the younger the bull, the easier and safer the job.

One such rodeo involved Fred Bewley, a farmer who kept suckler cows and their offspring. Fred was always immaculately dressed in a flat cap, sports jacket, collar and tie, and was an amiable gent. He was old school and very eloquently spoken. He had a competitive streak when it came to his stock, the prime specimens of which he liked to enter in local shows. Another thing about Fred was that everything he did was in slow motion. Everything. Even the speed at which he got his bulls castrated. You see, when you castrate a bull, you want them to be nicely grown but not too big, otherwise it becomes hard work closing the Burdizzo around the neck of a scrotum containing testicles that could be likened to small rugby balls. And just as importantly, it is also much more humane to carry out the procedure when the animals are younger because if the testicles are such a size, it is inevitably going to be more uncomfortable as they wither away once deprived of their blood supply.

Suckler cows' offspring generally can be hard to work with because the majority are born in the spring and have been out suckling and grazing for around six to eight months before they are brought in to be dehorned and castrated in the autumn. They are manageable but, needless to say, suckler bulls have had minimal handling and could kick like hell if something displeases them, such as a meddling veterinary surgeon. The trick was to stand sideways-on to present less of a target but this rarely prevents you returning home with your legs varying grades of black and blue.

Fred's bulls were a bigger problem, however, because he coveted the rosettes at the Auction Mart Christmas Show and so liked to have the biggest and best prize animals. In order to get his bulls into shape for the show he liked them to remain entire for as long as possible. The longer they had working testicles, the longer the testosterone would course through their bodies and the more muscle they'd gain. That was his theory, and it meant that each year, when called for castration and dehorning duties, we were faced with oversized beasts who were reluctant to be deprived of both parts of their anatomy.

Each year I would offer the same lament to Fred as I was kicked around by his prize bulls.

'You must get them done earlier next year Fred. It's not right leaving them until they're as big as this.' I even played the welfare card and explained that it was more painful for the bulls the longer it was left.

They were regularly between fifteen and eighteen months old and had testicles the size of mangos.

'They're too bloody big,' I muttered as I grimaced through gritted teeth, straining every sinew to close the Burdizzos on yet

Cock and bull stories

another oversized scrotal neck. Although the scrotums had been numbed, the patients still experienced a strange and unwanted feeling in their nether regions and consequently took this gross intrusion out on the vet behind and directly in the firing line.

Fred stood by watching me, looking slightly sheepish, sucking on the pipe that was always clamped between his teeth and which he removed on occasion, taking it out of his mouth and filling it with tobacco in slow motion, as if the effort was too much for him.

Fred spoke in slow motion too. He started a sentence.

'Aye. . .' he said, leaving the sound hanging in the air.

As I clamped the Burdizzos down on another sizable spermatic cord and got kicked on the side of the leg, I wondered if he was going to expand and offer any more.

'. . . and how's James?'

Changing the subject completely to enquire after the health of Jim Wight, my retired partner from the practice. He opened his mouth to continue. I waited.

'. . . I've not seen him lately.'

Fred then drew in a slow lungful of air through the pipe, and frowned when he realised that it had been so long between puffs that the tobacco had turned to ash. This was a common problem. For every ten pipes Fred filled with baccy, I estimated he managed to smoke one full pipe. The rest burnt away to nothing in the meandering fog he appeared to exist in.

'He's very good, Fred. Thanks. I'll tell him you asked after him,' I replied. A conversation about overly large testes was obviously out of bounds.

Tap. Tap. Tap. I looked over at Fred, who was methodically tapping the ash from the bowl of his pipe using a rung of the metal gate he was leaning on.

I moved on to the next patient, who again presented with a decently sized undercarriage. I sighed and shook my head.

Fred watched, and sluggishly filled his pipe with tobacco yet again while I was bent under the eighteen-month-old bull, trying to get a decent purchase with my Burdizzos.

Fred pressed the tobacco into his pipe in slow motion, placed it back in his mouth and continued his conversation.

'And Tim? Is Tim on good form?'

'Yes, Tim (my other partner) is good.'

He then reached into another pocket and pulled out a box of matches. At a snail's pace, he opened the box, took out a match and struck it. Even the strike was slow, so slow that the match flared against the side of the box and left a burn mark. As he raised it to his pipe the match spluttered out so the procedure had to be repeated. It was painful to watch. Fred seemed to be operating in another time zone to the rest of the world.

I sweated away under my patient while Fred didn't have a care in the world and continued his musing, warming up now and offering some gossip gleaned from his best mate, the local bobby, who was the font of all village rumour. As he recounted the story he stood watching me sweating and struggling to neuter half a dozen prize bulls. Each time I stuck a needle in to administer the local anaesthetic, they leapt up and down and jostled me against the bars of the crush, threatening to turn me into mincemeat at any moment.

Fred was completely oblivious to the frenetic activity and carried on chatting. He was a lovely man and I liked him a lot. Invariably, he'd invite me in afterwards to have a cup of tea and maybe a slice of cake. He and his wife had a cat which was very pampered and there was always something needed doing to her, whether she needed vaccinating or had a tooth that needed looking at or at the very least required worming. This was no mean feat at Fred's house. The cat always felt my investigations needed to be rebuffed at any cost, so I usually left Fred's farm covered in excrement, with a lacerated hand in addition to my bruises, exhaustion, and arms still quivering from the exertion of closing the Burdizzos on the oversized testicles.

As I mentioned previously, castrations can be done without local anaesthetic in the first week of life using elasticated bands, and so many farmers will do it themselves rather than pay a vet. The method is fairly simple but can be fiddly and you need to get it right the first time. It involves using a set of special pliers which have a head over which a strong rubber ring is fitted. As the head of the pliers opens, the ring, which is placed over the head, is stretched open. The scrotum is fed through the open ring, and when the pliers are released, the ring snaps back to its natural shape, cutting off the blood supply to the testicles. If the procedure works properly, the testicles will wither naturally. Sometimes, however, if it is not properly placed, one or both testicles may escape into the dangling scrotum above the ring, rendering the procedure useless.

This happened to Phil Shaw, one of our clients at Skeldale, who was a retired engineer, but who also had a smallholding on which he kept some livestock.

He called in shamefacedly, a few weeks after attempting the method on several of his calves.

'I don't want anybody to know this, but I dropped a clanger,' he admitted. 'I'm very embarrassed about it.'

Phil was a valued client and a friend, so I didn't judge.

'I thought I could castrate these calves on my own, but I haven't captured some of the testicles within the rubber rings.'

'So, it's gone pear-shaped?' I joked.

'You could say that,' he answered bashfully.

I went out to see what Phil had done and he assured me the bulls were ready and waiting for me in a corral he had rigged up, which he promised would make my life easier, cut the time I needed to carry out the procedure, and so reduce his bill.

'I know what you vets are like, you charge like wounded bulls,' he said.

Phil's idea of a good handling system and my idea of a good handling system differed somewhat. His ramshackle assortment of wooden hurdles tied together with string were dismantled within seconds of me appearing, so my assembled group of patients were back back with the rest of their mates in the main pen before you could blink. It could be described as a free-for-all, and Phil, who has a good sense of humour, did concede that perhaps he should have stuck to his day job. His pride was slightly hurt, having made a balls-up of the balls-off and cocked up the handling system, so naturally, as befits the Yorkshire character, I make sure to rag him about it whenever I have a suitable opportunity.

Castrations aren't everyone's cup of tea, and although they are painless for the animal, a lot of people get queasy around the subject. In one episode of the TV show *Springtime on the Farm*, at Cannon Hall Farm, I paired up with the actor Dominic Brunt, who plays vet Paddy Kirk in the ITV soap *Emmerdale* and whom I have got to know quite well. Paddy accompanied me to Cannon Hall, where a couple of calves required castration. The castration technique commonly employed at Cannon Hall involved removing the testicles surgically by incising into the scrotum with a scalpel. It was obvious that while Paddy was a lovely chap, he knew virtually nothing about animals or handling them. The fact that he's been marauding as a convincing vet for decades is a testament to his acting skills.

'The trouble with you is you spend all your time drinking in the Woolpack and you get nothing done,' I joked as he shied away from the business end of the calf with a grimace on his face.

In no time, I had administered local anaesthetic, had opened the scrotum with my scalpel and had removed two relatively small, glistening gonads with a quick twist and a pull. Paddy stood watching.

I couldn't resist when I noted Dominic's discomfort and queasiness.

'Can you put your hand out for me, please?' I asked.

When he did, I dropped them onto his outstretched hand. They were still warm. His face was a picture. He opened his mouth to speak but no words were forthcoming. He didn't know whether to laugh or scream. Now he really did have something to talk about in The Woolpack!

Regarding castration, it is generally the men who get squeamish. When couples home a puppy and come in for vaccinations and advice on flea treatment and worming, it's not unusual for the woman to ask how soon they can get their puppy castrated, while the men will say, 'There's no rush; let's talk about this when we get home. Is it strictly necessary, Peter?' It's almost as if it's an attack on their own manhood.

It is the personal choice of the owner, and in some cases, I believe there are valid medical arguments against castration. Some dog breeds, such as Labradors and retrievers, are prone to weight gain when castrated because their metabolism slows and because we often overindulge ourselves and our pets, leading to obesity. Lugging that extra weight about puts extra strain on their limbs and can lead to joint problems as they age. Hence, if I'm asked for advice, I will take each case on its merits. It may sound sexist, but there are clear medical reasons to neuter a bitch. It statistically reduces the likelihood of mammary cancers and eliminates pyometra (a nasty womb infection) in later life. Spaying also has the advantage of preventing unwanted pregnancies and prevents them coming into season twice yearly.

If a male dog becomes hypersexed and is pestering other dogs, humans, or cushions, for that matter, that is a valued reason to get the dog neutered. Dare I say, this is more common with some of the small breeds, especially Yorkshire terriers, which are notorious for it. I don't know whether it's the Yorkshire character; I'd like to think not!

Despite their propensity for amorous behaviour, I am a big fan of the Yorkie, and over the years I've had quite a following of Yorkshire terrier breeders, in particular, one lovely lady in Thirsk called Jenny Langhorne, who was a very well-thought-of Yorkshire terrier breeder and who sadly passed away at a very young age as a result of cancer. She was lovely and she had lots of mates from the Northeast and across the country who also bred Yorkies. They all shared advice and really knew the breed inside out. They were quite a community and often they'd know more about the breed than us vets. I have often said the Yorkshire terrier is very small in stature, but massive in character. They are quite unique. On many an occasion in the consulting room an owner will admit: 'He's very naughty with his cushion, you know, he's always humping it.' And I'll look down and see this little fella standing on the table who looks the epitome of innocence and appears to be saying: 'Me? No, no, no. You've got it all wrong. I would never do that.'

In a case which we filmed for *The Yorkshire Vet*, a woman who was on holiday in Thirsk made an emergency appointment because her dog had an erection that wouldn't subside and it was making the little chap quite distressed.

A dog's penis has a bulbous gland along the shaft which helps them tie with a bitch when mating. They can stay tied in sometimes for up to three-quarters of an hour. Sometimes the dog will dismount with his willy still inside, in which case the pair stand side by side until nature takes its course. The bulbous gland of the dog in question would not retract back into the preputial sheath. It is not uncommon and in such cases a vet often has to lubricate around the gland and manually push the penis back into its sheath. Sometimes we must sedate dogs in this condition because the act of just handling the penis arouses them even more.

One of the more unusual sex-based cases I've encountered happened recently when an owner brought her very sorry-looking bulldog in to see me. She was from Teesside and had made a real effort to dress up, with her hair pulled tight in a ponytail. She wore a figure-hugging small black party dress, which left little to the imagination, and furry sliders. She looked like she was on her way to a nightclub, rather than a trip to the vets. Her dog, she told me, was passing blood in his wee and she was very concerned.

'He's hurt himself down there,' she said, pointing.

'How'd he do that?' I inquired.

Suddenly she was quite coy.

'Well... You know. He's getting that way now,' she said awkwardly.

Trying to help her out I interjected.

'Do you mean his hormones have started to kick in?' I asked.

She took a breath, as if she was about to reveal a dark secret.

'He went out in the garden, you know. I was watching him from the kitchen window. I noticed there was a hedgehog on the lawn that took his fancy. He was quite interested in it, you know. Before I could get out to him, he started trying it on with the poor thing.'

The obvious jokes about feeling a small prick flashed through my mind but I said nothing. This was no time for joking. The poor dog had traumatised his todger while making an unwanted pass at an endangered species.

Instead, I raised an eyebrow.

I inspected him carefully and was pleased to see that his penis was fine, but his sheath was swollen and bleeding and had become infected.

'He's obviously had quite a go at Mrs Tiggy-Winkle because it's quite a mess down there,' I observed.

Thankfully, the damage was not permanent, and I cleaned him up, put him on some antibiotics and anti-inflammatories, and sent him home. He must have learned his lesson because I didn't see him again.

Hormones and hormonal changes cause just as many problems as they do for humans when they go out of kilter. I once treated a boxer dog called Bison who had a type of tumour in one of his testicles that produces oestrogen, which caused him to take on female characteristics. He developed breasts and his nipples massively enlarged. To coin an old Yorkshire phrase, they looked like chapel hat pegs.

Testicular cancer in dogs is not quite the concern that it is in humans where it can be extremely nasty and risks metastasising and spreading elsewhere. That's much rarer in dogs, and removing a cancerous testicle from a dog is usually curative, as it was with this patient.

Another boxer, Boot, came in one day with his owner, a long-standing client and friend named Steve Kendall, who is a joiner and carpenter. Boot had a mast cell tumour developing on his scrotum. Mast cell tumours can spread elsewhere and should be removed. When you do, you always treat them with respect and give the area around the mass a wide berth because they often spread into seemingly healthy surrounding tissue. They also release histamine

Cock and bull stories

into the surrounding tissue, which causes swelling and delays wound healing afterwards. This all meant that Boot's scrotum had to go in its entirety, along with his testicles.

The operation was a success and Boot, minus his manhood, never held a grudge. Dogs just get on with life, and whenever he came into the surgery afterwards, he was always pleased to see me and gave me a typical face wash with his huge boxer tongue.

But of all the sex cases I've encountered in my career, the one that sticks in my mind occurred way back in the Kirkgate years and involved the Greens, their herd of dairy cows, a prize bull and a sexually transmitted disease, which is rarely seen nowadays.

You may be surprised to learn that animals can carry venereal diseases and pass them around just like humans. This becomes particularly problematic if the carrier is a stud bull. This is what happened in the Greens' case, or at least it was according to their version of events. And it led to quite a scandal in the local farming community and a long-running feud.

It concerned a condition in days gone by called vibriosis, but to give it its correct name, is known as Bovine Venereal Campylobacteriosis (BVC), which causes infertility and abortion. It is spread by infected bulls when they mate susceptible cows and heifers. Once infected, a bull remains an asymptomatic carrier for life unless treated. Often the only way a farmer will know that their cows and heifers have been infected is if conception rates drop or if they have stillbirths. As farmers often rented out their bulls in days gone by to service herds on other farms, an infected bull could spread the infection widely and do a huge amount of damage.

I was called out to a farm that adjoined the Greens' land to look at one of their bulls which had seemingly developed fertility issues. The farm was developed by Lawrence Barker and by that time had been taken over by his son, John, and was run like a show farm. They had pedigree, high-genetic-worth stock. People used to come from all over the country to look at the Barkers' set-up. Their cows would give vast quantities of milk relative to many other dairy herds of the day.

After my investigation I diagnosed the bull with BVC. The treatment to cure the condition involved washing the bull's sheath out with streptomycin, a particular type of antibiotic. Like most farm veterinary work, it was not glamorous and involved a lot of back-breaking work under the bull, squirting the liquid into its sheath and then working it in and rubbing it along the length of the inside of the sheath to get on top of the infection. This needed to be done several times at weekly intervals. I became quite well-acquainted with the underside of that bull, and I can't be sure, but I think he was quite pleased to see me when I turned up. He never complained anyway, which was just as well as he weighed well over a tonne, something I was always mindful of when working away underneath him.

The Greens became involved when their cows were not in calf. I tested the cows and the results from the laboratory confirmed that they also had BVC. Although it could never be proved, Mrs Green maintained that the Barkers' infected bull had escaped his field, jumped in with her heifers, had his wicked way and infected them. The Barkers had a different slant on it. They claimed that when their bull got out, he was clean and that he caught the disease from one of Jeanie's cows, because, in true venereal fashion, it can be passed the other way.

Relations between the two neighbours were always frosty after that, and many years later, after John had retired and moved away, the Greens felt they had finally got justice of sorts. The Barkers' farm and its land, on the east side of Thirsk, was derelict but still owned by the family. Thirsk town spread out over the years as new houses and developments were built, but the development stopped at the Greens' boundary because despite being offered several million pounds for their land by a developer in the early nineties, the Greens refused to leave. It was the Greens' stubborn resistance that broke the chain of the development plan.

Stephen had lived there since 1944 after his parents moved there from Whitby. Jean always says that it would kill him if he had to move, so they weren't going anywhere. No amount of money would persuade them. Their determination to stay put stopped the next tranche of development east of Thirsk happening, because if the Greens had sold their farm to developers, it would have created a domino effect and the next available piece of land up for developments would have been that belonging to the Barkers. So, thanks to Jeanie's inflexibility, the Barkers were unable to sell their land for development and missed out on what I assume would be a considerable sum of money. As it stands at present, the developers have given up their plans to develop that side of Thirsk and have now moved on to other parcels of land around the town which are less troublesome. The Greens have created their own Green belt.

Revenge, as they say, is a dish best served cold.

10

'Ow do, pet?

Woody the 'micro' pig turned out to be more than his owner Diane bargained for. When she got him, around seven years ago, he was no more than a foot long from snout to tail.

'He won't get any bigger,' she was promised.

It transpired several years later, however, that Woody, who was a Vietnamese pot-bellied pig, was a giant among micro pigs. In fact, at around four foot long and some 80kgs, you could say he was a macro pig. Diane had been sold a pup.

Woody lived with Diane and her family. Her parents, Dave and Andrea, ran the fish-and-chip shop in Thirsk, which Lin and I visit on a regular basis. They were often called upon to organise Woody's care when Diane was at work.

One evening, when my wife Lin stopped by to pick up our tea, Andrea asked her if I'd get in touch or drop round as Woody needed some attention.

'There might be some free chips in it for him,' she offered.

This discussion was held over the sound of the bubbling fryer at the chip shop and Lin explained to me that Woody needed his feet clipped. It transpired later that in the din she'd misheard and it was actually Woody's teeth that needed attention, which concerned me, knowing the damage they can do.

For a red-blooded Yorkshireman, the offer of a free dinner was too tempting to refuse, however, and I ventured along to meet Dave, who was pig-sitting that afternoon.

I've explained before about my reservations about treating pigs and Woody was no exception, particularly as he had some form in this respect, having previously raked his tusk on a cameraman when he was being filmed for *The Yorkshire Vet*. He could be quite a force to be reckoned with and I approached the task remembering an anecdote of Alf Wight's about a farmer he knew who was gored in the groin by a pig.

'Aye. He went in with that sow. Bye she wor nasty and she had a right go at 'im,' he recounted. 'She let one of his pebbles out.'

With those words ringing in my ears, I pulled up outside Woody's house. He lived in a chest-high wooden enclosure in a pig-secure run in Diane's back garden, and Dave met me by the gate.

'Are you feeling strong, Dave?' I asked.

'Not really, why?' he asked quizzically.

'Because I need you to hold Woody's mouth open while I see to his tooth,' I explained.

Dave, who was familiar with Woody's temperament and strength, did not relish the thought of being at the sharp end of this particular pet.

'You're alright, Peter, thanks,' he declined. 'I'll leave it to the expert.'

I was joking of course, and it transpired that the job was more complicated than a quick piece of dentistry. Woody's left tusk was so long that it had curved into his cheek. It was tricky to get off and he needed to be sedated by injection to get him off to sleep.

We coaxed him into his indoor chalet, lifted the lid off so I could lean over, and Dave held a board against the opening so he couldn't escape. I managed to administer the intramuscular sedative, with Woody squealing his objections as only a disgruntled pig can. Once we had sedated him, we let the rather grumpy Woody out to wander around the garden while we retired to a safe distance and waited for the sedative to take effect.

I was pleased phase one of 'Operation Woody' was out of the way. Dealing with pigs in farm conditions was never easy, and dealing with pigs in people's back gardens was not my idea of fun.

It was a warm, sunny day and after ten minutes Woody was gently snoozing in the sunshine, snoring away. I knelt to check on him and when I took hold of his tusk to have a better look, he struggled and grumbled. 'He may be off his feet, but he's not in a state that I can work on him,' I explained. 'He'll need a little longer.'

Ten minutes later he was finally out for the count, and I had a proper look at his teeth. The long tusk was of particular concern because, as I had feared earlier, it had started growing into his cheek and would have started to cause him some pain. I had to work fast because he was a big lad and there was a danger that he would be awake in no time. As I've said, sedating farm animals in the field is not an exact science and you can be lulled into a false sense of security by a slumbering patient.

The plan was to saw off around four inches of tooth with a cheese wire. The tooth was curved back so far into the cheek that I couldn't get the wire between the tooth and the flesh, so instead I had to feed it through the curve of the tusk. Once I'd done that it only took a few quick saws back and forth to cut through the

'Ow do, pet?

first few inches of tooth. It was so quick I had time to get more off and managed to get the tusk down to a much more manageable size and out of the way of Woody's cheek. He grumbled a bit as I continued to pray he was firmly in the land of Nod.

All the while Dave stood over me watching while I was on my knees, ready to make a hasty retreat to a safe haven should Woody rouse from his slumber.

With the tusk dealt with I started on his trotters. The back claws were quite long and when I snipped the first one, Woody jolted. My heart skipped a beat and I got ready to make a dash. But the sizeable boar grumbled and went back to sleep, allowing me to complete his pedicure, or should I say piggycure. Job done, I left him lying in the garden snoozing, glad to get away with all my fingers and limbs intact, looking forward to claiming my chippy reward. The things you do for friends!

Woody was one of the more unusual pets I saw on my rounds and not necessarily the type of animal you'd expect to see in a back garden in the suburbs on the outskirts of Thirsk. But as the old saying goes, *there's nowt as queer as folk* when it comes to choosing pets. I've learned over the years that what would have seemed unusual decades ago when I started working as a vet, has now become commonplace.

Take hens, for example. When I was a youngster a lot of people in the village kept hens in their gardens for eggs and occasionally for meat. But habits changed, food became cheaper, people had more money to spend and less time, and the chicken and egg production industry became more intense and more industrialised. By the time I qualified as a vet in the eighties, it would have been rare to see a normal household with a chicken coop in the back garden. All the chickens were in battery farms or in large deep litter sheds.

But then people started to become more aware of animal welfare matters and started taking in, or rescuing, liberated battery and intensively reared hens, or hens that weren't productive enough for the demands of modern farming. So now it is common to see people with hens in the garden again. It's even become a thing for people in towns and in the suburbs. And I can see why. It's a lovely thing to be able to look out of the window and see hens scratching about, pecking a little morsel here and there. It's very therapeutic for people and the hens benefit too. For me, it encapsulated the ideal relationship we have between animals and people. It should be a two-way street. It shouldn't just be about us getting benefit from the animals, the animals should gain as well. With hens that have been taken in from battery farms, it's a win-win situation because those birds would have been destined for slaughter otherwise, and instead they get to live happy lives.

It is also important to have an understanding of farming practices. Many will assume that intensively reared chickens lead a miserable life, and some do. But not all. Indeed, some have a pretty good life. People often look at outdoor animals in the middle of summer when they're running around the countryside, and in those conditions then life is good for the animal. But they don't see them in the middle of January when they're wading about in mud and they're cold and miserable. Chickens in intensive situations in those conditions are arguably better off as they have warmth, shelter and food and are safe from predators. I'm not defending one or the other, and as a vet, my concern is always the welfare of the animal. What I am trying to get across is that there is nuance. It's not always black and white.

Pets go in and out of fashion. Like hens, ferrets used to be commonly kept when I was younger, because people used to go

'Ow do, pet?

rabbiting. And while people still do, it is a dying pastime, largely because tastes have changed and rabbit isn't a commonly eaten meat anymore. Now, if someone has a ferret, it's more likely to be a pet. We had several clients at Skeldale with pet ferrets. One lady used to take hers out for walks on leads around town. One of them was called Honeyball Lecter and I treated him once for a case of mites, which proved quite hard to diagnose. His name was a play on the terrifying character of Hannibal Lecter in the film *Silence of the Lambs*, played by Sir Anthony Hopkins (who also played Siegfried Farnham in the 1974 feature film *All Creatures Great and Small*, based on my old boss's books). When Jodie Foster's character in the movie entered the high-security prison to interview Lecter, the scene wouldn't have quite the nerve-jangling impact if Jodie's character, Clarice Starling, greeted the famous psychopath with the words: 'Hello Honeyball.'

Rarer types of pets can prove more of a challenge to treat, as was the case with a coughing baby peacock who was brought in by his owner. We don't get many pet peacocks in North Yorkshire. This youngster had been adopted by a man who had a caravan at a site in Thirkleby, the village I was born in. He'd found the peacock when it was a chick. It had been abandoned by its mother, so he took it in and raised it. He was rightly proud of having rescued the chick and reared him into a healthy little bird. The little fellow had 'imprinted' on him (meaning that the youngster regarded him as a mother figure) and followed him around everywhere. It used to waddle into his caravan and sit with him and his wife watching telly in the evening.

It took me a while to work out what the problem was but the strange type of cough the peacock was exhibiting gave it away. He was suffering from a parasitic disease called gape worm. In this condition, the male and female parasites pair up and attach themselves in the host's trachea. They produce eggs, which the host then coughs up and swallows. Once in the digestive system the eggs hatch. The cough presents as a gasping or snicking noise, as if the patient has got something stuck in its throat. I treated this young peacock with a particular wormer, and he was in full health in a few days. He was a pleasure to treat.

People have asked me in the past if there are any species I don't like dealing with, and if I'm honest, I'm not good with snakes. This isn't due to any phobias. It's because you can't read a snake. You have no idea what's going on inside a snake's head. You can have a snake on the table, and you look at those eyes and they are just totally impassive. You can't tell a thing about how it's feeling or what it's thinking. A dog wears its heart on its sleeve; you can tell everything about them by their demeanour, the look in their eyes, their ears and their tails. Cats will let you know what they are thinking by the way they swish their tails or raise their hackles. But a snake is just one long, expressionless tube with two blank eyes and a tongue. I never know if a snake is in a good mood or not, so generally, if I'm called on to look at a snake, I'll refer it to a reptile specialist who knows about these sorts of things.

That said, I have treated snakes before. One client in the distant past had two pythons and many years ago he brought one in to the surgery because it had stopped eating. The first challenge was examining it. Fortunately, the owner was an expert at handling his pet, and as he held it from above, supporting its body, he moved his hand to the jaw, and as the mouth opened I could use a pair of forceps to open the mouth and peer inside. The diagnosis was staring back at me. It was suffering from a condition called mouth rot, or infectious stomatitis. It is common in lizards and snakes when they are under stress and caused because the immune system weakens and fails to keep the bacteria normally present in the mouth in check. One of the treatments used in those days was an antibiotic called metronidazole, which we had on the shelf for treating cats and dogs. I gave him the treatment, confident that it would be curative and that it was a job well done.

He went away, and a week later he was back with a second snake and some bad news. Snake number one didn't make it. On those damning words, my confidence took a heavy blow.

'I'm sorry to hear that,' I consoled. 'What seems to be the problem with this one?'

'I think it might have the same condition,' he explained. 'It's off its food.'

Once again, I managed to coax the reptile's mouth open, being careful of the fangs, and examined the oral cavity. Sure enough, there were the tell-tale signs of mouth rot, albeit this time not as bad as the former patient. Again, I treated it with the recommended medicine and sent him away, slightly less confident than I had been the first time.

A week passed and I came in one morning to the practice and flicked through the daybook. There was a message from the snake owner. Two words.

Python died.

It upset me. Those were two animals I'd been unable to save. Results like that knock your confidence. I churned it over and over in my mind. The diagnosis was correct. The treatment was correct. So why did they die? These are the types of cases that torture veterinary surgeons on a daily basis, and I made a mental note for the future to pass any more of these difficult creatures onto colleagues with greater expertise in reptiles than I had.

About six months later, a chap rang up and wanted to make an appointment because he also had a snake which was off-colour. He specifically asked for me, which puzzled me. Frankly, I wasn't sure whether I could help or not. And I wondered why he chose me. After all, my track record with snakes wasn't great to say the least. I would of course do my best, but why me? So, when he came in with the snake (which wasn't a python), I asked him.

'Do you mind me asking why you specifically wanted to see me?' I inquired. To be honest I felt quite nervous. The previous experiences had shaken my faith in my abilities.

He replied: 'One of my mates had two pythons that you saw and he recommended you.'

I thought for a moment.

I frowned. 'The gentlemen who had the pythons with mouth rot?' I asked.

'That's him, yes,' the man replied.

'But they both died!' I exclaimed.

'Yes, I know,' he said, 'but my mate said you were the snake expert.'

Some expert! It highlighted to me just how unpredictable snakes can be. These owners knew their animals and realised that when they became ill there were no guarantees they would recover, even with the correct diagnosis and treatment.

This was illustrated by the recent case of Snakey. His owner, Andrea, who also owned oven-glove-devouring Wesley, brought him in because he was constipated. Fortunately, at the time, we had a young Portuguese vet working with us, Sarah Abreu, who was very interested in zoo work and, although inexperienced, knew quite a lot more about snakes than I did. Initially I gave Snakey some medication by mouth to try and lubricate the suspected faecal build-up, but it wasn't effective, and he came back a few days later no better. We had concerns that if there was a total gut blockage, any impaction could cause the overlying gut to die off. We took the decision for Sarah to operate on him. She discovered that the pressure of the impaction was indeed causing the bowel to die off. Sadly, however, Snakey didn't survive the op but would have died anyway, so he was given the best chance.

Unfortunately, operations like that on exotics are very hit and miss. These creatures are very sensitive, as owners know. In order to keep them healthy, everything needs to be just right as we try to mimic their natural habitat, nutrition, environment and routine. I believe that these animals need to be looked after by experts to ensure their welfare requirements, as well as their environmental and behavioural needs, are met. And even when those are all correct, things can still go pear-shaped very quickly.

Not that dogs and cats aren't still prone to the unexpected. In North Yorkshire we have a lot of working dogs, and they generally get quite excited when they're out on a shooting day where they'll work side by side and often all pile in a trailer together along with their owners to be taken to where the shoot is taking place. In this situation they'll be in very close confinement, sitting there, excited about what they're going to do, panting, tails wagging, anticipating the joys to come. In these conditions there's a greater risk of passing on certain infections from one to another, such as kennel cough, which can be a problem because it is so infectious. If you have fifteen dogs in a trailer and one is coughing, it is quite likely that they will nearly all catch it, and suddenly the practice will have a rush of dogs who've been on shoots being brought in to be treated or to be vaccinated to prevent it from happening. There is nothing like these flare-ups of infection to focus owners' minds on preventative medicine.

Sometimes we see patterns of disease for other reasons. For example, we see isolated cases of Weil's disease, which is often spread through rat urine or a rat bite. Cases are often fatal despite modern supportive treatment, and so when there is a case, especially involving a fatality, the practice in the following weeks is often inundated with requests for vaccinations from owners whose dogs' vaccination programmes have lapsed.

People and their relationships with their pets never cease to amaze me. They do become part of the family, and often, an owner's relationship with their companion animal will be as important, if not more important, than their relationship with their friends, or even their husbands and wives.

Sometimes those relationships are much more than just companionship and people rely on their pets, particularly when the animal is a service animal.

In Thirsk, Dave and Linda were a partially sighted couple and they both had guide dogs which they worshipped. I'd known Dave for years. Dave was a dead keen fisherman, and he knew that my dad sometimes used to organise fishing trips off the coast of Whitby, so he'd chat about fishing when he came in with his dog. As he was partially sighted, his other senses were much more acute, and he was pretty good at catching fish because he would feel movement on the line better than an able-bodied angler. He was a lovely chap. You never saw him get down or depressed. He was always laughing and joking and full of life. I used to see him and Linda out in the marketplace with their white sticks, arm-in-arm with a dog on each side. It was remarkable the way they manoeuvred themselves around like a single unit, people and dogs working together in perfect harmony. Dave knew everyone and could recognise people by their voices and pick them out, even in a noisy shop or street.

The dogs came in for six-monthly checks and would be wormed, vaccinated and weighed. Their feet and nails would be checked. Every point of health was examined. The Guide Dog Association issued each dog with a booklet which would be filled out to ensure that everything was meticulously recorded, because these dogs had to be kept in tip-top health. We didn't charge. We did it because those dogs were vital to their owners' lives. It used to be a pleasure to see them and put the world to rights with Dave and listen to his fishing tales and other stories of joy.

Dave and Linda were not the sort of characters to let their disability prevent them from living life to the full. While their guide dogs lived with them, other owners of service animals are supposed to maintain a more professional relationship with theirs, although that's rarely the case because we can't help but get attached to the animals in our lives. Skeldale had a contract to look after North Yorkshire Police's dogs. Some were quite aggressive and would have to be muzzled by their handlers before we could check them; others were big softies. And although I don't want to simply generalise, the dogs were not supposed to live in the houses of their handlers. They were supposed to live outdoors in a kennel, and they were definitely not supposed to go inside the home, sit on the sofa and watch television with their handlers. I can't say for sure, but I suspect that was not always the case. I suspect some of those dogs may have crept in and been given such treats more than just occasionally.

They were phenomenally well trained, as I discovered after Skeldale got broken into some years ago. One of the vets had arrived to a patient on a Sunday evening after dark and was unlocking the back door and keying the password into the alarm system when it went off. At exactly the same time, some ne'er-do-wells were at the front of the building smashing through the glass entrance and raiding the reception. The vet called me and I told her to get back in her car, lock the doors and stay out of the way. I called 999 and raced to the practice, and by the time I got there, the police had arrived and the thieves had gone. All the crooks could find were collection boxes on the reception desk for various animal charities, which they made off with. The police had dogs, which were given a scent from the reception to work with. They shot off across several fields and, using their amazing powers of scent, managed to find the empty boxes about half a mile away. I found this canine detective work quite incredible.

They are so intelligent, and their sense of smell was so finely honed, it was a privilege to see them in action. Like I always say, I see a lot of dumb people, but I don't see any dumb animals.

One of the other jobs I did for North Yorkshire Police was to assess its horses when the horseback section was disbanded. The stables were based at Harrogate, and it had been decided that because the region didn't have any big crowd events to police, the horses were surplus to requirements. I was asked to go and value them. It was a very sad job to do because it was obvious how much the mounted officers were bonded to their horses. They were best mates. The Irish police, the Garda, were interested in taking some; others were destined for the Cleveland police force.

I'll never forget that visit, going from horse to horse. By the side of each one stood its rider, who was losing their partner and best mate. Several of them tried to nobble their horse's chances in the hope that the animal would be put out to pasture and that they would be able to keep them themselves.

'He's not good in traffic; there's no point in him going anywhere.'
'This one's clumsy around people.'
'He can bite a bit, given half a chance.'
'This one doesn't like being close to cars.'

'Ow do, pet?

The excuses kept coming and I fully understood why.

Human and animal relationships are as rich and varied as human–human relationships. They say we are a nation of animal lovers and in my experience that's true. Most people want to do right by their pets, their livestock and even the animals they work with. Which is why people often ask me whether there are things they can do for their pets to help them feel comfortable when they need to visit a veterinary practice. There certainly are, although some animals are never going to enjoy the experience. That's just the way they are, in the same way humans vary in the way they feel about going to the dentist.

The main thing is to try and keep them calm and not give them reasons to get upset. Unless they are regular customers, most pets go to the vets every once in a blue moon and so the veterinary waiting room and examination rooms are unfamiliar environments with strange smells and sounds. And let's face it, nothing really nice happens to them in a veterinary practice.

Some people will bring their pet's favourite toy with them, so they have something familiar. It is also a good idea if the pet is coming in a carrier to put their blanket or bedding in there with them so they feel at home.

Pets do get attached to their toys in the same way humans do. Even King Charles III reportedly still keeps his favourite childhood teddy bear, as it was recently revealed. Our cat Toddy has one that he really loves. It used to be a woolly sheep, given to me by British Wool for some promotional work I did for them, but now it's just a tattered ball of wool that Lin has repaired so many times there is more cotton in it now than wool. No matter that it's falling apart, he carts it about the house with him, and wherever he's sleeping, we'll find his favourite sheep.

If an animal is in to stay, it is doubly important to take in a blanket or bed from home and some toys. Some owners will bring in a piece of their own clothing because it has their scent on, which is another good idea. Pets like familiarity, calm and quiet.

When Skeldale was being designed we deliberately created a long waiting room so that people could sit in a row not facing other owners and pets, but looking out at the pet food stands opposite. We did this because at 23 Kirkgate the waiting room was a square sitting room with chairs all the way round the periphery, meaning that for the animals, all the other animals were in view. There could be a greyhound looking at a cat in a basket on one side and a rabbit on the other. Skeldale also designated one end of the waiting room purely for cats, which we felt was a good idea to keep them calm.

Anyone who owns, or has owned, a cat will know that they have complicated relationships with other cats and can easily get upset by the slightest change in their environment. Mrs Smith, a true feline lover and client at Skeldale, had two cats. One was called Basil and he was the archetypal gentle giant that wouldn't say boo to a goose. He looked a formidable character at first glance, but if truth be told he was one of the biggest softies I have ever come across. One day another cat appeared in the neighbourhood and started to venture into Basil's garden. Basil became utterly neurotic. He refused to go outside, even though he was twice the size of the intruder. On the odd occasion Basil did pluck up courage to risk going outdoors, one sight of his nemesis and he would bolt back indoors and take refuge upstairs under his owner's duvet, shaking like a leaf. It was such a small change but poor Basil's life was tormented once this potential bully came on the scene, so much so we had to put him onto long-term anxiety-reducing medication.

'Ow do, pet?

In our house even the appearance of a suitcase will trigger our cat Toddy's neurosis. He'll think we're going away and try to climb in the case in the hope he can come with us. Suitcase packing signifies turmoil in Toddy's routine. Although there are plenty of lovely catteries around that take good care of their guests, for cats, which are very territorial and love routine, it's probably a difficult experience. All cats would rather be at home where they are surrounded by familiarity.

If pet owners do decide to have more than one cat, or dog for that matter, early socialisation is important for them to develop the skills they need to cope with their housemates. Dogs that live in a single-dog household should still be introduced to other dogs at an early stage so they can learn how to behave and react when they meet others on their travels.

It's a vet's job to try and keep his patient calm, which is a skill I learned over the years. In my younger days I sometimes met force with force. If, for example, I had a stroppy bull I'd grab his nostrils and say: 'Right pal, if that's the way you want it, that's the way you can have it.' I could tell from the animal's eyes whether they were going to be aggressive or whether they were frightened, and adjust the way I approached them accordingly. But I would also have to watch for changes in behaviour, because fear can sometimes lead to aggression.

Some animals, on the other hand, are ideal patients and treat an encounter with the vet with a degree of resignation. They look at you as if to say: 'Just get on with it.' Others are timid or anxious and need support and care and understanding. Then you have the patients like Possum, who are just out-and-out aggressive and want a scrap, come hell or high water.

And then, of course, vets have owners to deal with, who can be equally as demanding or nervous as their pets. I've always lived by the saying, *Do unto others as you would like to have done unto you*, so if a client is polite to me, I will be polite to them, and if they are brusque with me, I tend to be brusque with them. In the vet world, we deal with so many different characters, from the aristocracy to people who live very basic, simple lives. I like to think I've always had an ability to get onto their wavelengths, associate with them, understand them and understand the type of veterinary service they want. If someone is getting a bit tetchy about something, I can spot it a mile off. If someone's unhappy with the type of service I've just suggested, I can see it in their face. They don't even have to say anything. And I'd like to think I'm pretty good at getting on with people and liaising with them. As a vet, I know I'm never going to be able to save every animal or cure every ailment. But what I can do, is do right by my clients. Alf Wight helped instill that in me.

One day I was down in the dumps because I was unable to save a cat. Alf Wight noticed my glum demeanour and asked me what the matter was.

'I've seen Mrs Henry, and her cat's going to die. There's nothing I can do about it,' I said.

'Remember this, Peter,' he said. 'You can only do your best. If you've done your best, no one can ever question you. But you must always do your best.'

And I've often passed that advice on to young graduates and trainees. It is part of a vet's responsibilities to take ownership of each case. Even though you have to remain professional, you can't help becoming emotionally invested in cases and taking it personally when some do not work out. Those words of Alf's are always at the back of my mind. If you haven't done your best, it's not been good enough.

11

My life in pets

I'm going to say something controversial. Young vets make some of the worst dog owners, in my opinion. That might sound harsh, or even shock some people, but it's based on what I've witnessed over the years. It's not because vets are in any way cruel, negligent or irresponsible. Far from it. No, the problem with younger vets often is the hours the profession requires them to keep. Working in a veterinary practice and owning a dog are generally incompatible because dogs enjoy company, plus a regular exercise routine, and veterinary life does not lend itself to routine. Veterinary practice often requires long, unsocial hours.

Many vets and vet nurses do get dogs, and some make it work, but I've always made it a point to caution younger staff and assistants over the years because dogs are a big responsibility. I've known vets to take their dogs with them to work and leave them cooped up in a car for hours on end when they are working, and it's really no life for your beloved companion. Many years ago, one vet who came to work at Skeldale bought a Jack Russell terrier pup, against my advice. She took her out with her on visits, which was fine, but then she was locked alone inside the car for hours on end when the vet was working in the clinic. I fully understood why out of sheer boredom she entertained herself by chewing the upholstery and seatbelts to pass the time. One day I caught a glimpse of her handing the little dog over to Jim Wight because she couldn't cope with her. Jim's daughter, who worked from home, had kindly offered to take her.

There are exceptions but unfortunately, generally speaking, single vets haven't got the time to devote to dogs, especially in mixed veterinary practices. That's the truth of the matter, in my opinion, and is why I didn't have dogs until later in my career when Lin was at home and my life was more settled.

Instead, when we first got married and Lin was working full-time, we had cats, because it is true cats are much more independent and are happy to be left on their own at home, coming and going as they please through a cat flap.

The first cat we had was called Zak. He was a lovely fellow, but one day he went out and never came home. Sadly, that's not uncommon and has been the fate suffered by many a cat lover, who loses a beloved pet and never gets the closure of knowing what happened to them, whether they came to grief on the roads or whether they were enticed away by someone else who fed them better cat food. Cats can be fickle creatures and don't always show the loyalty their owners would like. When Zak disappeared, we put signs up on the lamp posts and pictures of him on noticeboards around the area but there were no sightings. He vanished and we are none the wiser to this day as to what happened to him.

Over the years in my career, I have heard of numerous cats disappearing without trace like Zak. Many owners, rather than accept that their pets may have been run over, cling to what I would call conspiracy theories. In these theories, shady characters drive around at night stealing cats from neighbourhoods. I dismissed these rumours as fantasies until one morning when a couple whose cat I treated called in to Skeldale ashen-faced. They were 100 per cent reliable characters and responsible cat owners. I had no reason to doubt them. They explained that the previous night they were looking out for their cat to return home from her usual evening stroll when they noticed a small dark Peugeot car pull up just past their house. A lady got out, picked up their cat and bundled her into the back of the car, which drove off at speed, never to be seen again. I was horrified that such events were actually happening.

In the mid-eighties, after losing Zak, Lin and I went to a cat rescue centre in a village just outside Northallerton which was run by a lovely lady who was what people would today call a typical 'mad cat lady' – somewhat cruelly, I might add. She was devoted to the animals in her care and wouldn't turn a moggy away, no matter what state they were in or what their chances of being rehomed were. She was obviously scrimping and scraping to keep it all going and lived in a bungalow with an ever-revolving colony of kitties. I discovered that she was also highly protective of those under her care.

When we turned up unannounced, a young couple, she eyed us suspiciously. I am lucky to be able to quickly assess people's thoughts and feelings and I got the distinct impression she thought we might be unreliable pet owners.

'What are you looking for?' she asked.

'Well, we'd like a cat, we don't really mind what type,' I said. 'We've usually had boys, but we don't mind girls.'

She went into one of the back rooms and brought out a fierce-looking feline, whose hackles raised on viewing us two trespassers. As she stroked him, I could hear a low, rumbling growl emanating from his throat.

'This one likes being outside,' she said. I took that to mean that he was semi-feral and would be off on his travels at the first opportunity.

'They'll be living in the house quite a bit,' I said politely.

Her eyes narrowed.

'Do you know much about cats?' she questioned.

'A bit. I'm a vet,' I replied.

In an instant, her demeanour changed. Her icy exterior melted and she almost skipped with joy. She plopped the grumpy cat down on a chair and it scarpered off with a parting grumble.

'Why didn't you say? I have some kittens if you'd like one of them.' She grinned.

Until that point there had been no mention of kittens. We had been upgraded.

'We'll certainly have a look,' I said.

She went into another room and came back with two lovely ginger kittens, full of life and meowing away. Suddenly, I could do no wrong and her guard came down completely.

'These two are brothers,' she said. 'Which one do you want?'

I looked from one to the other and then at Lin. I could tell we were both thinking the same thing. How could you choose one over the other?

'Do they get on with each other?' I asked.

'Oh, yes,' she replied. 'They're inseparable.'

Well, that made our minds up for us.

'We can't choose; can we take them both?' I asked.

The lady was only too pleased to let us have them both and was delighted that her kittens were going home with a vet.

And that's how Rodney and Rupert became our first pets as a married couple. They were lovely characters and very different, considering they were brothers. Rupert was very intelligent, a bit

My life in pets

standoffish and very agile. Rodney was as thick as a plank, but very loving and very clumsy. We had just moved into our first home, which needed a lot of work, and were a typical young couple at the time, hard up and saving gradually to do up the house. We had one expensive carpet in the hallway. Throughout the rest of the house we had to make do with cheap ones. Rodney and Rupert decided at a very early stage of their residency that they didn't want to go out and pee, they wanted to pee in the house instead, but they didn't want to use the litter tray, or even the cheap carpets for that matter. They chose the hall carpet. The nice one. I used odour eliminator, stain remover and anything else I could think of in the hope that removing the smell, or masking it, would discourage them. It never did. Eventually, a large chunk of our expensive, but ultimately stinking and discoloured hall carpet, had to be replaced.

We loved having Rupert and Rodney but sadly, they didn't have long lives. We got them in the days before commonplace testing for feline leukaemia, which was, and sadly still is, a common viral infection in cats, so owners never knew for sure whether their cats were carriers. When they were around six years old their mouths started to get very sore. Their gums became increasingly inflamed, as they developed severe gingivitis. These were common symptoms of feline leukaemia, and I feared the worst and tested them. The results came as no surprise when they came back positive. The virus destroys the immune system in a similar way as HIV does in humans. There was no treatment. We had to keep them away from other cats because the condition is contagious and is passed on to other cats through bodily secretions, such as saliva, which can easily pass to an adversary in a cat fight.

Their condition deteriorated and I felt helpless. Their mouths filled with ulcers and every mouthful of food would feel like eating fire, but in the early stages I was able to control the inflammation through long-acting corticosteroids, painkillers and antibiotics. Lin and I both knew what was coming. There was only one outcome, and so when Rupert got to a point where it wasn't fair to keep him alive anymore, I put them both to sleep at the same time. I made the decision, and as I was not at work that day, I called the practice and asked someone to come and carry out the dreaded procedure for us. It was a busy day, and I waited several hours, in which time I fully understood the emotions people go through when they decide to put their pet to sleep and wait for a vet's appointment or visit. As an owner, you watch the clock tick down, lamenting every minute that passes bringing you closer to heartache. After three hours I told Lin I was going to put them to sleep myself. And that's what I did. They drifted off peacefully together, finally out of pain and at rest. Over the years I've often thought of those sad last hours spent knowing what was to come, and I've said to many of my clients that once you make the decision to put an animal to sleep, don't wait. Just get it over with as soon as is practically possible, for their benefit and for yours as well, because it's torture waiting.

For some years after that we didn't have pets. Life became busy. Work on the house progressed, but it was always my intention to have animals and, having grown up around dogs and cats, I always knew that one day we'd have dogs too. After our children were born and Lin was permanently at home, it just seemed right that a dog or two would complete the family.

For some time, I'd liked boxer dogs, despite having reservations which stemmed from an incident when I was a young vet. I knew a chap who owned one and the dog's favourite trick when he attended the practice was to hold out his paw to shake hands, and when you went to shake, he'd go for your hand. It made me quite wary of boxers. However, again early in my veterinary career, a boxer breeder named Sue Green moved to Thirsk and became a client.

Sue was one of the top boxer breeders in the country. She had forthright opinions and didn't suffer fools gladly. Below that tough exterior, however, was a heart of gold. What she didn't know about boxers wasn't worth knowing. This is a trait I've discovered again and again in my career. Breeders and owners often have an in-depth understanding of their own animals, and I used to tell visiting students that we do well to listen to them. I can't understand some vets who have the mentality that only they know what's wrong with the animal and sometimes completely dismiss the observations of a worried owner.

I used to have long chats with Sue about her boxers. She was fanatical about the breed. Her dogs were top class despite the fact that she bred dogs with slightly longer muzzles. This meant they could breathe easily, unlike short-muzzle breeds nowadays, which are quite rightly frowned upon by my profession. For many of them, breathing normally is a massive and sometimes impossible undertaking.

I fell in love with the boxer character. They wear their hearts on their sleeves and their emotions are always amped up. If a boxer is sad, they'll look like the world is on their shoulders and slump around with droopy eyes as if a cloud is hanging over them. But if they're happy and excited they bounce around like Tigger from *Winnie the Pooh* and can't contain themselves.

I became friendly with Sue, and very early on, before I was married, she offered me one of her retiring stud dogs called Simon. I couldn't dedicate the time needed to give him the life he deserved so he went to live with Sue's mother in Devon, but even then, I always thought one day the time will arrive when I can have my own boxer. Nevertheless, at the time I felt highly honoured that this sometimes ferocious lady would consider me a worthy owner of one of her top dogs.

Many years later when Lin and I had started a family, one of Sue's bitches had a litter. By that point we had decided we wanted the kids to grow up in a household that had dogs, in part to teach them how to respect and care for animals. I spoke to Sue and she introduced me to Bert, a small bundle of energy and joy wrapped up in a brindle boxer puppy body. I couldn't resist, and at eight weeks of age Bert came home with me.

From the very start, Bert saw himself as one of the children. He had to join in with whatever it was they were doing, and if he couldn't, he would pull what we called his 'boxer face', which was a hangdog sulking expression. He hated being left out. The kids loved having him around. They would dress him up. He would jump on their skateboard and have a go himself. They had a pull-along cart too, and he'd jump in with them, on top of them, when I was pulling it along the garden, until it was just a tangle of human and dog limbs. If they were playing a board game he'd sit there watching intently, as if he was trying to work out the rules. He used to drive them crackers at times because if they were playing with a ball, he'd think the game was just for him, snatch it and run off with it. Whatever you threw for him would never get brought back. He'd just take it and scram. The kids would be calling Bert! Bert! Bring it back. And he would be off somewhere in the distance, standing forlornly there, looking at them, wondering why he'd been excluded from the game. He really didn't have a clue what he was doing. I suppose he wasn't the smartest dog in the world, but by God he was fun.

Not a day went by when we didn't crease up laughing because of something or other he'd done. His mannerisms were hilarious. When he got excited about something, he'd snort like a boxer in

My life in pets

training, bounce up and down on all fours and then stop, and then look at me quizzically as if to say, 'What were we going to do? I forgot. I was excited.'

His mannerisms and expressions were priceless. If Bert was told off, he would look at you out of the corner of his eye, huff and then go and lie down somewhere with his tail between his legs. It was so funny. He looked like a sulky teenager. We always knew exactly what mood he was in. He used to have an indoor kennel in the house and if he wanted to get away from the kids, that's where he'd take himself for some peace and quiet.

He loved his walks, usually with Lin because I was at work. We were living in Thirlby Village then, and Lin and Bert would go up the lane towards Donald Sinclair's house and take a big circular route where Bert loved to spend hours sniffing around, seeing which other dogs had been there and left their scent, which he would then pee over to leave his calling card. He would stop around twenty or thirty times to do that, by which time there was very little coming out. Such are the pleasures of being a male dog.

When visitors came, Bert always had to say hello. All he wanted was to be loved and to join in, which, to me, is what defines a boxer.

Bert could also be a sensitive soul. One of my mates, Tim, lived in the village further down the road. He was a farmer, and his land was set back behind his house. One day Lin was taking Bert for his walk; they passed Tim's front gate and his farm dog came out from the entrance and went for Bert. He didn't do a lot of damage, but it upset poor old Bert, and up until we moved three years later, every time we got to the end of Tim's drive, Bert would have a nervous look to see if his attacker was there lying in wait. He never forgot, and although it never happened again, Bert wasn't taking any chances.

Bert was active and healthy. He had a few minor health problems that needed intervention. For example, when he was just over a year old, he developed a small lump on his leg – a histiocytoma. These are common and benign skin masses that can sometimes clear up on their own, but when this didn't, I removed it surgically. A few months later, he developed a lump on his side – a mast cell tumour, which was much more concerning. I removed it and made sure I also removed a wide margin of tissue around it. It was sent off for testing, which confirmed it was a medium grade tumour so would have been likely to spread to the surrounding tissue if not removed in its entirety.

Although when I operated on him, I concentrated on the surgery and remained calm and professional, in the back of my mind there was always the thought that this was my boy on the table and I had to look after him because he was relying on me. It made me appreciate even more what people went through when they left their animals with us for operations. They were entrusting a member of their family to us, and that confers a huge responsibility on us to make sure we do the best we can, just as Alf Wight always used to say.

Bert recovered from his surgery, albeit after a slight regression when the wound opened. But I fixed that, and later in life I had to carry out another minor procedure on him when he developed a condition called epulis, which boxers are prone to. Epulis is an overgrowth of the gums that present often as small cauliflower-like growths. Epuli can get quite big and can ultimately grow over the teeth. When Bert's started to affect how he was eating, I took him into the practice to trim the growths off and take his gum margin back under general anaesthesia. If I'd have had such an operation on my gums, I would have been on huge amounts of painkillers and reluctant to eat for days afterwards. I fully expected Bert to behave in the same way. However, despite what sounds like horrific surgery, when he returned home he insisted on eating his dog biscuits.

Boxers are also prone to something called cardiac syncope, which are fainting attacks. You could be going along as usual on a walk, the dog will get excited, and all of a sudden they will stop and keel over. It looks terrifying. The faint only usually lasts for half a minute and they then come round, stand up, shake themselves off and carry on as if nothing has happened. It happened twice to Bert. Once after Lin took him home from having his stitches out after the tumour surgery. He'd been in the car and got himself all excited, and when Lin arrived home with him, he collapsed on the driveway. She called me in a panic and I rushed home, but by the time I got there Bert was fine and running around as if nothing had happened. The second time it occurred was when I was training for the New York half marathon. Bert came with me on my runs, and he fainted on one of them. Again, after a few seconds he was as right as rain. I like to think that I was putting in such a good pace that he fainted with the effort of trying to keep up, but I think in reality Bert was having an off day.

Several years after we got Bert, I was driving through Thirsk and noticed a small bundle of fur by the side of the road. I slowed and looked at what I realised was a small kitten trying to cross. I pulled over, ran back and picked it up. It was a tiny little thing and looked ragged. I could feel its ribs through its long, tortoiseshell hair. It was obviously a stray. I took it to the practice where it was warmed up and checked over. Being a tortoiseshell, the cat was obviously female. In the following days she made herself at home, got her strength back and left quite an impression on all the staff, including me. We made inquiries to discover if there was an owner, but no one claimed her, so I took her home. Lin and I named her Rosie.

She was a lovely cat and settled in immediately. Having lived on the streets for the first months of her life, I'm sure she knew which side her bread was buttered. Bert wasn't that impressed, as she soon established herself as the boss. If he was in the wrong place on a chair or bed she fancied, Bert was sent packing with a little tap of the paw, not necessarily with claws protruding. It was hilarious to watch. She would strut up to him, brazenly pat him as if to say, 'Off you go then', and he'd let out a sigh, get up and skulk off. Just like me, he knew his place in the pecking order.

To us, however, she was very affectionate and would seek out a warm comfy bed or lap and happily snuggle up to be made a fuss of. She'd often follow Lin when she took Bert out for his evening walk, trotting along, twenty yards behind, past the village hall, where Bert always chose to poo, hiding in the darkness because there were no streetlights. It made a wonderful sight, Lin in her nightie and dressing gown, searching out Bert's deposits to be bagged and removed, Bert sniffing and peeing, and Rosie darting through the shadows.

Years passed and Bert matured into what in dog years would have been his adulthood. He was still prone to excitable outbursts but mellowed, as happens to us all.

Sue came in to Skeldale one day and mentioned that she had another litter and that one of the pups, a male, was available, should I be on the lookout for a companion for Bert. Now, I had always believed dogs are very sociable and enjoy the company of other dogs, which in the most part they do. As Bert was more mature now, and as there was no sign of a friendship between him and Rosie (except on Rosie's terms), I thought it might be a good idea to bring another dog into his life. Lin and I had always discussed having another, and we decided that we would take Sue up on her offer.

My life in pets

Alf came to live with us just as we moved into a new house which had land and required lots of building work. He was a beautiful red colour, but otherwise almost a clone of Bert in terms of behaviour. He was just as much of a livewire and had all the boxer traits that Lin and I had fallen in love with. Bert, however, was not as impressed. He was starting to slow down at that point, and I think, in hindsight, maybe he just couldn't be bothered making an effort. Alf was full of enthusiasm and wanted Bert to be his mate. He was a young whippersnapper who wanted to play constantly. Bert, on the other hand, was in the pipe-and-slippers period of his life and just wanted to take things easy. It was at that point I started to question whether dogs really do always like having other dogs about, especially when it comes to coping with divided attention from their owners.

But to his credit, Bert put up with Alf, and eventually they worked out a pecking order and grew comfortable with each other, although for the rest of his life, I could tell that Alf liked Bert more than Bert liked Alf.

They were very similar. Neither of them were castrated because they showed no interest in what Lin used to refer to as 'that dirty business'. I think they were both asexual.

To us they were both extremely loving and loyal. They both adored being with the kids. Alf, too, needed to know exactly what was going on around the house. When we were having the building work done, we had heaps of soil at the front of the house by the road and Alf would climb to the top and sit there all day, keeping an eye on the people and cars that passed by. He was incredibly nosy. If he had been a human on a housing estate, he'd be what you'd call a 'curtain twitcher', spending hours at the window, engrossed in the comings and goings of neighbours and desperate for a bit of gossip.

He'd pester the builders the whole time to play. As far as he was concerned, they were just there to entertain him.

There was a cottage attached to the house, and if people stayed, Alf would always wander in when they opened the door in the morning, looking to see if he could get a second breakfast, or just to be nosy.

We chose not to take the dogs out anywhere in the car because they would get too excitable. We tried once to take them to the seaside, but it was hell. They never settled in the car and got themselves so worked up, panting and drooling everywhere, that we vowed never to do it again.

They weren't the most obedient dogs, which is embarrassing for a vet to admit. We did try to train them but failed miserably. They just didn't have the attention span. There was always something more interesting that needed further investigation. Any commands of recall were met with deaf ears.

They were both friendly with other dogs, Alf particularly. He loved every dog he met and wanted to say hello and have a good old sniff. If we were out walking and he was off the lead and saw another dog, he'd be off, turning a deaf ear when I called him back. I'd run after him and often found him sniffing around a worried-looking owner, whom I'd have to assure that he was just being friendly. Some of the male dogs took exception to his exuberance and they'd have a go at him. Alf was quite offended by this. He didn't take social cues.

When Bert was ten, he developed a cough which didn't clear up after a few days, so I took him into the practice and X-rayed him. There was nothing apparent on the X-ray image, and when the cough persisted, I carried out an endoscopic examination of his throat and upper airways but couldn't find anything to suggest the cause of his cough, which was worsening week by week. I tried all sorts of things. I tried antibiotics. I tried anti-inflammatories.

I tried cough suppressants. But the cough persisted and I became increasingly frustrated, not knowing what was causing it. It didn't seem to be bother him too much, but after about another month or so we noticed specks of blood as he coughed. This was very serious, I feared. Up to that point I hadn't considered that it might be a malignancy. He was still quite bright and he wasn't off his food or losing weight. Once again, I booked him in for more X-rays, and Lin brought him in to Skeldale one afternoon. I asked Tim, my partner and colleague for thirty-six years, to help me. I sedated him, X-rayed him, and when I saw the image my heart sank. It showed a big cancerous mass on his right caudal lung lobe which was very obviously growing quickly.

I had very limited options. I could have done a thoracotomy and removed the lung lobe with the mass in it, but lung cancer in dogs never ends well. It might have bought him a few months, and he was ten years old at that stage. Boxers, sadly, don't make old bones.

It was a heartrending decision and one I was in no frame of mind to make. Lin was with me. We were both distraught.

'It's not good news,' I said with tears in my eyes as I showed her the X-ray image. 'What are we going to do?'

We were floored. We were not expecting it.

'I can't do anything for him,' I said. 'Let's just take him home for a few more days and think about things.'

Lin, to her credit, was the strong one.

She took a breath to steel herself.

'No,' she said, 'we're going to do what's right for Bert.' And I knew what she meant by that. 'There's nothing we can do, so it's better and kinder to put him to sleep now, while he's here.'

I had spent my professional life advising people that once they had made the decision to put their animal to sleep, not to delay.

Do what's best for the animal, not what's best for you, I told them. Don't prolong suffering. Yet, when that decision knocked on my own door, I came up lacking, and as I say, it was Lin who was the strong one, who realised it was the right thing to do.

I tried to clear my head of emotions and thought about the last weeks. I thought about Bert, trotting across the field at home, coughing as he went. He wasn't ill but his cough was getting progressively worse, and I'd seen enough of these cases to know that in the very near future there was only going to be one outcome. His condition would worsen quickly, or the tumour could impinge on a blood vessel, which then could rupture, and he'd have choked to death on his blood. I couldn't take that risk. He'd got to ten and a half years old. I'd seen boxers go on longer than that, to twelve or thirteen years, but a lot of them don't live to a ripe old age. They're not the most robust breed from a health point of view. Even without the lung mass, he was unlikely to live a long life. It was not right to struggle on to the bitter end. If I took him home, I was taking him home for my sake, which was wrong. Over the years I'd seen people keep their animals going for their sake, not for the sake of the animal, and in that moment, I fully understood why they did so, but I knew Lin was right. We had to let Bert go there and then.

The last thing I did for Bert – my boy, one of the family – was to put him to sleep. Lin and I, choking back tears, stroked him and made sure he knew we were there with him at the end. He died peacefully, having lived a full and happy life. We were bereft.

Over the following days we came to terms with the loss and carried on with our lives. It was a busy time at home, where we were still having major renovation work done on the house, half of which was a building site. Life had to carry on, and Bert was always there, living in our memories and always on our minds.

My life in pets

Every now and then we'd find one of his toys or another artefact to be reminded of him, which brought a mixture of joy of having such a wonderful dog and sadness that we had lost him.

Both Alf and Rosie knew. Alf would often sniff around and then whine, having picked up Bert's scent from around home. To our surprise, Rosie seemed to take it hard too. She was never a particularly demonstrative cat, but when we came home without Bert that miserable afternoon, the builders were still there doing the groundwork on a part of the house which at the time hadn't been built. There was a gap between the habitable part of the house and the unbuilt new section. Rosie hated the builders and the noise they created and never ventured past the gap. But when she realised Bert had not returned with us, and maybe sensing our sadness, she walked across the gap, across the building site, yelling and howling as she approached us. It was the most out of character, unusual behaviour I'd ever seen her exhibit. It was as if she was howling with grief. And the next morning she came upstairs to our bedroom, yelling again. She just knew part of her family was not coming home again. How did she know?

One of the realities of having pets is that generally we outlive them and so have to grieve for them when they die.

Some years later, Rosie's health began to deteriorate too. With her, I noticed a mental and cognitive decline. Her behaviour started to change. Whereas previously, she always steered clear of Alf's bed and preferred her own spaces, I got up one morning and found her in his bed, with him sitting by, looking quite perplexed and a little put out. She always went outside to go to the toilet, but she started to go out of the back door, look around in confusion, come back in and then do her business on the hall carpet. It was totally out of character. By that point she was old and was displaying the classic signs of dementia, which I have witnessed several times in aging patients. Her mental decline was mirrored by physical decline. She became very arthritic and her back became weak and stiff. She struggled to walk. One morning we came down to the kitchen and I saw that she was in a really poor state; she'd gone from her bed into Alf's (which she never normally did) looking very sad and forlorn. I knew it was time, and took the decision to put this bundle of fluff I'd rescued eighteen years earlier to sleep.

Although we had Alf, who was still in his prime, the house felt incomplete without a cat and so it was always in the back of mind to get another. The opportunity came a while later when the RSPCA brought a middle-aged moggy in for a check-up. She was around eight or nine years old, a nice-looking cat but with major health problems. She had seizures and heart problems and had lived a tragic life to date. She had lived with a hoarder whose house had burned down and she had been saved from the fire. We discovered that she loved ham because seemingly that's what she had been fed on. She was called Mary, and as she had nowhere to go, I decided that with all her problems, she must have a home with me.

Alf accepted her with grace, and she became part of the family. She enjoyed the trappings of home life and would come and sit with us in the evenings in the living room, her on one side of the sofa, Alf on the other. Occasionally she'd be sitting on a cushion on the sofa, have a short duration seizure, fall off, recover and then climb back on again.

In 2010, I received news that shook my life to the core. Lin was diagnosed with breast cancer, and I didn't know how to cope. I was terrified I'd lose her, and while she faced the battle and the treatment with fortitude and strength, I crumbled like a wet biscuit. When she was ill, Mary and Alf sensed it, and they became a great comfort. Lin would be on the sofa, ill after chemo and surgery, and Alf would come and put his head on her knee and look at her as if to say, 'I'm here for you.' He wouldn't play up at all. Mary would sit there as well. The truth be told, they were fonder of Lin than they were of me. I was just the bloke that turned up from work, but they shared their lives with Lin. I used to say to clients when we were talking about the bond they had with their pets that if Lin had to choose between me and the dog, I'd have to pack my case because they were so close. Lin was a a god as far as they were concerned, and when they knew she was ill, they supported her through her treatment and recovery, sometimes, I felt, better than I could.

Alf was a healthy dog and only had one or two niggles up until he was nine, when he developed a lump in his neck. It was one of his glands. Dogs can get a condition called lymphoma, which is a form of malignancy which I'd seen and treated frequently during my career. I checked him regularly to see if any other glands had enlarged, but none did. However, the size of the sub-mandibular gland slowly increased, and I made the decision to take it out. I had to pluck up courage to do so because it was tricky surgery near several major blood vessels and nerves. I performed the procedure myself because I could not put that responsibility onto anybody else in the practice. The surgery went well, and I sent the sample off for histology. The results that came back made my heart sink. Alf had lymphosarcoma, a cancer of the lymph nodes, which are storage sites for white blood cells and a vital part of the immune system. I hoped that I'd caught it in time and that it hadn't spread. It was promising that no other glands had been affected, and after that I regularly checked all his other peripheral glands. It became a force of habit when I was petting him, feeling around his neck and under the tops of his legs and other regions where lymph nodes can be palpated easily for any tell-tale lumps. None of them ever came up and he never showed any signs of being ill. And after several months I breathed a sigh of relief, thinking that maybe we'd got away with it, that we'd been lucky. That was the only operation Alf ever had and I told myself that Alf was a robust dog.

A year later, when he was just turned ten years old, our luck ran out. Andrew, my son, was home. I had popped home at lunchtime to do some work and have a bite to eat. It was a routine part of the day and Alf knew that after I went back to work just before 2pm, he'd be taken for his walk, so at around 1.45pm he would come and find me and start nudging me, as if to say, 'Off you go, it's time for my walk now'. You could set your clock by him. He'd get excited and run and get his lead, dropping it at Lin's feet.

On that fateful day I went back to work at the usual time after the usual reminder, and Alf, Lin and Andrew went for their walk through Kilburn Woods opposite our home. Alf was prancing about as normal. He saw one of his mates, a black Labrador, and bounded over to say hello. They had a run around together, as they always did, and Alf, as usual, was full of beans. They were out for around an hour and took their usual route. Like his owners, Alf was a creature of habit. Together they came back to the road and walked a few hundred yards back to the house when Alf collapsed suddenly in the driveway. His legs gave way, and the next thing Lin and Andrew knew, he was lying on the ground, panting, barely conscious. Lin called me immediately. I could tell straight away from the urgency in her voice that something serious had happened.

'I'll be there in a few minutes,' I said. I raced to the car and thankfully there was little traffic, so I was there in around ten minutes. I found Alf lying on his side with Lin kneeling over him. I went to him and could immediately see he was blue – the medical term is cyanotic, and it means the blood is not being oxygenated. I listened to his heart; it was about 170 to 180 beats per minute, and it should have been about 120. His heart was racing to try and get oxygenated blood around his body. It could have been acute onset cardiomyopathy. I didn't know and I ran back to the car to see if I had any drugs that would help. I didn't but I knew we had some injectable heart medicine back at the practice that could help. Alf seemed to be hanging in there.

'I'm going back to Skeldale to get something,' I told Lin, and I hurtled back down to the surgery, raced in, grabbed what I needed and raced back out again to the car. On the drive back I got stuck behind a vehicle, the owner of which I think was out for a leisurely scenic tour. It was impossible to pass on the narrow country lane and I sat behind impatiently, tailgating in a desperate effort to get the driver to hurry up. The drive seemed to take an eternity. When I got back home for the second time, Alf was still breathing but he wasn't in a good way. I whacked the drugs into him and prayed.

'Come on, Alf,' I willed. 'Please don't leave us.'

Minutes hung heavily, time slowed. His breathing became increasingly erratic. His eyes fluttered. His breathing slowed. After a few minutes, it stopped. Alf died in the driveway, in front of us. We were stupefied by the suddenness of it. We were shell-shocked, stroking him and staring at his body that just half an hour previously had been an animated ball of energy playing with his mate in the woods.

I've played that day over and over again in my mind. I don't know if he'd have died anyway or if I would have been able to save him if I had been able to administer the medicine a few minutes earlier. I'll never know the answer. The probable cause of death was a massive cardiac incident, the reason for which will elude me to my dying day.

As we stood there, stunned, Lin went inside and brought Mary out to see him. She didn't want Mary to go through the unexplained loss that had upset Rosie so much. She wanted Mary to understand what had happened, that her companion had died and not just disappeared. She looked at Alf pensively. She understood.

The following weeks were awful and empty. Again, I busied myself with work, leaving Lin with the hardest part, being in a house without Alf. I could escape; she was surrounded by memories. Three weeks later, it got worse when we had to put Mary to sleep. She had been having so many problems by that point. She'd always had problems with her joints, asthma and intermittent seizures, and things were getting worse as she got older. It was a difficult time. It seemed that in the blink of an eye we had a home with no animals at all.

Alf left a massive hole in our lives, and the manner of his demise seemed to make it worse. We didn't have time to say our goodbyes. For months on end afterwards, Lin wouldn't go into the woods with me for a walk because that's where she went with Alf and it was too painful to be back there without him. I've seen people suffer more when they've lost a canine companion than when they've lost a spouse and I can understand why. We still miss him. On the inside of our downstairs toilet door, there are some little specks of dried spray from when Alf had snorted once or twice on his regular visits accompanying Lin on her trips to the lavatory. Lin won't clean them off because that was Alf, and it reminds her. Alf's been dead since 2018, and those stains will always stay there for as long as we live in that house.

After a while, people began to ask us if and when we planned to get another dog. We don't know. Filming became busier and my plans to retire were put on ice when I moved to Grace Lane Veterinary Practice. Lin has her mother to look after who is deaf and virtually blind, and with things as they are now, it wouldn't be fair to take on another dog. Taking on a new dog is a massive undertaking because they need to get to know and trust you. But we never say never, and in the meantime, I've had the honour of becoming a patron of Boxer Dog Rescue Northern England, a wonderful charity based in Lancashire that we've visited on numerous occasions and which was featured on *The Yorkshire Vet*. It does wonderful work rehoming boxer dogs.

After Alf died, the house was soulless and I started looking out for a stray cat to bring home, because in the practice, people were always bringing them in and they'd often end up in rehoming centres or with the Greens, who have taken in numerous waifs and strays over the years. Cats fit in better at home presently because of our comings and goings, as they are more independent.

One morning, a chap came in to Skeldale wearing a fluorescent hi-vis jacket covered in oil. He had a little bundle of fluff in his hands. It was hard to make out what it was because it too was covered in oil.

'I've rescued this,' he explained and held out a kitten that was looking very sorry for itself. 'Can you do anything with it?'

Near the surgery there was a recycling centre called Todd's. He worked there and found this little kitten in one of the skips. How it had got there we'll never know. I checked it over and noted it was a little boy.

The nurses took the kitten away and started to clean him up. He was a good-natured little thing and had obviously been through quite an ordeal.

He needs a home, I thought to myself as I watched him getting scrubbed down with detergent.

I rang Lin.

'I've found somebody,' I said. And that lunchtime, when he'd been properly cleaned and dried and fed, I took Toddy home. He was so young he still needed feeding with milk, so Lin fed him four times daily.

Toddy, who would have been dead now if that kind young chap hadn't seen him, is no longer a helpless kitten. And is he grateful? Not in the slightest! He's quite selfish and very aloof. He likes his own company but he's a great character and a prolific mouser. He goes out, raking about all night, seeing what he can torture and kill, and then sleeps all day. He's a bit of a thug really. He doesn't like too much fussing and messing about; sometimes he likes a stroke, but it must be on his terms as he's not that affectionate. If he does let you stroke him, his belly is a no-go area and God help anyone who attempts to rub that.

He's a clever opportunist, as I discovered when I started feeding barn owls that live in the woods over the road from my home. Every night at dusk, I leave day-old chicks out for them. These are kindly donated by a nearby chicken hatchery. They are surplus to requirements on hatch days and are humanely euthanased. I always feel happy that their very short life hasn't been wasted and that they are a necessary part of the food chain. I place them on a platform on the front of my owl box, which I climb up to each night, using a ladder. Toddy often followed me out and I never realised why until I spotted him sneaking up the ladder and pinching a chick when he thought I had gone back indoors. I couldn't help but laugh, but I made sure from then on the ladder was taken down after I'd been up it.

Never underestimate the intelligence of animals.

12

Yorkshire, through and through

Mr Braithwaite lived on a council estate in Thirsk in the eighties and kept pigs in a few buildings on the Thirsk Hall estate. This was not unusual. Lots of people who weren't farmers in the traditional sense kept livestock to supplement their incomes and their larders. Mr Braithwaite was a client of the Kirkgate practice. He was a genial fellow, who followed what today would be classed as a very thrifty lifestyle. He didn't drive, he had a bicycle. He didn't own a phone either. If he needed to speak to a vet, he'd pedal into town, usually with a cigarette hanging out of his mouth, ash blowing back into his face. Like a typical Yorkshireman, Mr Braithwaite was direct and a man of few words. He told you what he was thinking and wasn't particularly diplomatic.

Mr Braithwaite had a recurring problem with his pigs. They were kept in small brick pigsties and occasionally, when the sows had litters, the piglets picked up an infection, and sometimes all or the majority of the new-borns died. The condition they had was called bowel oedema, which is caused by an E. coli bacterial infection. The illness, which is rare nowadays, causes swelling of the bowel walls and usually happens at the weaning stage. The poor piglets lose coordination and start to stumble around. The condition also causes fluid to build up in eyelids, which become quite puffy. It gives the impression that the piglets are sleepy, staggering around with half-closed eyes.

The best way of avoiding bowel oedema is good hygiene, but Mr Braithwaite wasn't a large-scale farmer, and in those days, power-washing stock buildings with disinfectant were not commonplace. Hence, the E. coli infection used to self-perpetuate in his buildings and became a constant problem for him. Regularly, he'd pedal up to the practice, dismount, come inside and explain: 'Me pigs got boweel edema.' He became quite fixated with the condition, and even when they didn't have bowel oedema and had another illness, he would diagnose it himself and tell the vet on duty: 'It's boweel edema, they've got it again.' The way he mispronounced it sounded almost sing-song.

Farmers would often mispronounce veterinary terms. For example, one day when one of Mrs Green's cows was overdue and needed to be induced, she called and said: 'Peter, she should be calving now. I want you to come and seduce her.' I wondered whether I should put on my best aftershave for her. Salmonella was also occasionally adulterated to a much more pleasant 'Simon Ella'. Another classic malapropism going back to Alf Wight's day was when a farmer called to report an outbreak of swine erysipelas, a soil-borne infection. 'I think I've got another case of that smiling Harry syphilis,' he explained.

Unfortunately for Mr Braithwaite's piglets, there wasn't very much we could do once the cases were established other than administer antibiotics and hope they recovered. They rarely did.

I'd not been long back at Kirkgate after my spell in Luton when I was sent out to one of Mr Braithwaite's latest litter of piglets, which, sure enough, had been infected with this particular strain of E. coli and were showing all the signs. However, a litter from the other sow he kept appeared to have dodged the infection and looked very healthy and were thriving. I gave the sick litter the usual treatment and hoped that it would work, but in the back of my mind I was extremely pessimistic.

A few days later I was leaving the surgery and saw Mr Braithwaite cycle past. I'd not heard from him as to how the piglets I'd treated were faring, so I ran after him, calling his name. He stopped further up the road near the church when he heard me.

'Mr Braithwaite,' I panted. 'How are your piglets doing?'

He looked at me and nodded.

'The piglets are doing nicely, thank you,' he replied.

It's fair to say that my heart lifted. The greatest compliment I could ever have was knowing that I'd been successful.

'That's wonderful news, Mr Brathwaite.' I beamed. 'It's always touch-and-go with bowel oedema. To be honest I doubted they'd make it.'

He looked at me, puzzled, and then a spark of recognition crossed his face.

'Oh, those piglets you treated,' he said, deadpan. 'They all died. But rest of 'em's aw right though.'

And with that he put his foot on the pedal and cycled away, leaving me standing there, quite stunned, and completely deflated having been brought plummeting back to Earth.

I recount this story because it perfectly encapsulates the type of no-nonsense character I have encountered throughout my career. But although Yorkshire folk aren't afraid to voice their opinions and may appear brusque to some, underneath beats a heart of gold and a warm hospitable nature. In Yorkshire, a brew and a slice of cake is social capital. There's many a Yorkshire housewife who wouldn't be out of place on television's *Bake Off*. There's a reason why the world's best tearooms, Bettys, are in Yorkshire.

As a vet in a place like Thirsk, you cannot help but become a part of the community where you get to know everyone. Through their animals I've been privileged to meet some wonderful people throughout my career who have become not only friends, but part of my family, for instance, people like the Greens. Rarely a day goes by when I don't speak to them. When you treat people's animals over decades, you befriend them and a mutual trust builds, and in a way, you become part of their extended family.

Another close friend is Rosemary Guthe, whose horse, Big Jim, and two dogs, Cracker and Drummer, were patients of mine. Drummer, a black Labrador, was a deep-thinking, intelligent dog, while Cracker, a yellow Labrador, was more like his name, a boisterous, enthusiastic fellow who did not share the intelligent traits of his father. Mrs Guthe was always very perceptive when it came to her animals. She'd research symptoms and come in and see me and explain what she thought the problem was. Inevitably, she was always correct, and when I prescribed medication, she would research that too, so that she understood exactly what it did and why I was recommending it.

Drummer developed heart problems and arthritis as he got older, so I used to see him regularly for check-ups. I used to look forward to it because Mrs Guthe and I would have long chats and she'd give me advice on many different issues. She isn't one for gossip and tittle-tattle. She is a very sharp, intelligent lady who has an undeserved self-deprecating nature. She speaks a lot of common sense, and our relationship developed to such a point that my wife used to joke that she was 'the other woman in my life'.

Yorkshire, through and through

The more I learned about Mrs Guthe, the more fascinated I was. She comes from a family who owned vineyards in Chile and she has cousins all over the world who are all hugely successful. One even has an airport named after him. She was an interpreter and can speak many languages very fluently. She's a talented musician and used to be the ladies' captain at Seaton Carew Golf Club. Whatever she did in life, she excelled. She married into a German Jewish family and her in-laws owned a shipping line that sailed out of Panama. Her husband, Digby, inherited the business and she launched some of the line's ships, which were built in Sunderland. She showed me a cork once from one of the bottles smashed against the hull of a new cargo ship. They owned a large estate on the outskirts of the town which encompassed several farms, a village pub and other assorted businesses.

Digby died when he was fifty-three, many years ago. They had a son who was sixteen at the time, so she had the unenviable task of keeping the estate going until her son was old enough to inherit it. Although she is what could be described as landed gentry, you just wouldn't believe it if you met her. She wears worn clothes and always tells me that she's slow-witted. But she's not. Underneath her unassuming exterior her mind is as sharp as a razor. I liken her to having an intellect like a cross between the TV sleuths Miss Marple and Columbo.

She's incredibly well-travelled and knows everything there is to know about shipping. Lin and I are partial to cruise holidays and Mrs Guthe always takes an interest when we book one. She checks out the seaworthiness of the vessel, when it was last in dock for an overhaul and looks at records to make sure the ship is well maintained. She is not interested in what she refers to as 'the domestic arrangements', meaning the luxuries of the cabins. She even checks out the captain, as she explained to me that British or Scandinavians make the best skippers.

In the early noughties, Lin and I booked a cruise which was due to pass through the Panama Canal, as this was something I'd wanted to do for many years. The cruise line we were going with was not scheduled to stop in Panama City, where Mrs Guthe had a cousin, Johnny.

'I'd love you to meet Johnny, Peter,' she implored.

'But Mrs Guthe, the ship doesn't stop in Panama City,' I explained.

'I'll see what I can do about that, Peter,' she said cryptically.

A few days later she came to the practice late in the afternoon, as was her habit. She waited for afternoon surgery to finish so she could have a chat and would invariably sit very patiently in her car until consultations were concluded.

'Peter, I've made a friend I think,' she said. 'I've asked Nigel at the cruise line if we can stop the ship in Panama City and he's going to think about it and get back to me.'

The 'friend' was one of the directors of the cruise line, who she'd been in touch with. I'm ashamed to say I was a little sceptical. If I'd personally made that approach and request, it's fair to say the person at the other end of the line would have thought I was a lunatic and hung up.

A week later she came in to see me again.

'Nigel's been on the phone. He's going to stop the ship at Panama City now when you go on your cruise next year.'

Sure enough, when we checked out the itinerary, the ship was making a stop in Panama City. The cruise line had never stopped there before and to my knowledge has never stopped there since. It's a working port and it's quite difficult to get people out of the port area to the taxis at the gate.

Yorkshire, through and through

Nevertheless, on our cruise it stopped in the port and Lin and I, along with around 800 other passengers, went to explore the city. We also met Johnny, who was delightful and who we've met several times since when he has been in the UK visiting Mrs Guthe.

Wherever we went on our ports of call, Mrs Guthe would recommend places.

'If you're in Cozumel, you must visit Pancho's Backyard; I think you'll like it. They make the best margaritas in the area,' she said with a smile and a twinkle in her eye.

Sure enough, we found Pancho's Backyard, which from the front looked like a hardware shop but had a beautiful terrace at the back overlooking the ocean where they served margaritas in glasses that were as big as goldfish bowls. How did Mrs Guthe know this? When we left Pancho's Backyard an hour later at 11.30am I had to return to the cabin for a snooze, such were the size and potency of Pancho's cocktails.

When we went to Singapore on another cruise for our silver wedding anniversary, she told us to go to Raffles Hotel and have a Singapore sling. It sounds as if Mrs Guthe is a big drinker, but she's not.

'There will be a girl behind the bar at the hotel who will come out with a tray of them already made,' she said. 'Tell her you want to see one made in front of you. You want to watch them make it.'

Raffles is the world-famous hotel in Singapore named after Sir Thomas Stamford Raffles, accredited as the founder of modern Singapore. The hotel that bears his name is very exclusive and was frequented by many of the hierarchy of the British empire. One of the traditions when you have a drink in the famous Long Bar of the hotel is to have a bowl of monkey nuts and discard the shells onto the floor.

Sure enough, when we went to Raffles in Singapore we were presented with a tray of readymade cocktails, as Mrs Guthe described, so we asked to see them made instead of drinking a pre-made one. We were then treated to a display of mixology. Being a Yorkshireman, I'd already noted the prices of the cocktail and so to get value for money I wanted to see how it was concocted.

At the time of writing, I've known Mrs Guthe for over thirty years and we've had long chats and Sunday lunches together. She's in her eighties now and treats me somewhat like a surrogate son. She's a formidable lady and a valued friend. This is the kind of the relationship that you sometimes have with the people whose animals you treat throughout the years. Her character also typifies the Yorkshire persona. Common-sense, straight-talking, sharp and hospitable.

While Mrs Guthe and Mr Braithwaite represent different facets of the Yorkshire persona, certain animals also represent Yorkshire traits, such as Yorkshire terriers, which are physically unassuming but tenacious and are apt to make their opinions known.

I've had the pleasure of meeting and learning from some of the world's top Yorkie breeders, such as the previously mentioned Jenny Langhorne, who taught me so much about the breed. In my early career at Kirkgate I carried out one of my first caesarean sections on one of her bitches, and the puppies needed to suckle. I was very tentatively trying to coax one of the puppy's lips onto the end of the teat when Jenny exasperatedly took it from me and she said: 'Peter, don't do it like that. You're being far too gentle. Look, get the mouth open, grab the teat, and latch it on so the teat is going down the back of its throat.'

She thrust this puppy onto the teat she was holding between her thumb and forefinger, and it immediately started drinking.

'That's how you do it,' she said.

One of her other tips was to put a bit of butter on the teat too, because that gets them to latch on, she'd say.

Yorkshire, through and through

She, like many other breeders, had all these snippets of invaluable knowledge. Her dogs were shown at Crufts and all over the UK, and before shows she'd sometimes bring them into the surgery adorned with 'crackers', which are squares of tissue paper attached to the coat and held in place with elastic bands to prevent the hairs from trailing on the ground so as to stop them getting dirty and broken. I likened it to a woman in bygone days having curlers in her hair before going out socially. I suppose that's one of the similarities of the human and animal worlds. It sometimes requires a bit of indignity in order to look your best later.

'I see they're dressed in their teabags, Jenny,' I'd joke.

One of the best places to see Yorkshire people and their animals has always been the Great Yorkshire Show, an annual event in Harrogate that brings together everything that is so special about my part of the world. Although it is primarily an agricultural show, and the largest in the country, it is so much more. It provides an opportunity for farmers and local businesses to show the world what the region has to offer. I've been going there since I was a child. It holds a very special place in my heart. Being a Yorkshireman, it gives me an immense amount of pride because it epitomises so much that makes Yorkshire great and how much Yorkshire has to offer.

I have a well-developed routine whenever I visit, which has been a habit for as long as I can remember. Firstly, I make a beeline for the cattle. There are dairy breeds such as Holsteins and Jerseys, as well as traditional British breeds such as Shorthorns and Herefords and many of the continental breeds such as Charolais and Limousin representing the crème de la crème of cattle. For me, as a child, seeing all these animals was like being a child in a sweetshop. Now, when I go and follow the same routine, it is amazing to see how these breeds have changed over my lifetime as the quality of the progeny continues to be improved. It is a privilege to stand and gaze at the best of the best of breeds on show, and I think of all the work and decades of careful breeding and selection that have gone into producing the magnificent creatures we now see.

Next, it's the sheep and all the different, fascinating breeds. I didn't realise as a youngster there were so many types and that they were so magnificent. The other thing I have always been interested in is the rare breed enclosure at the show where you can see some of the breeds that are under threat of dying out and even close to extinction. It is here that I learned how the Rare Breeds Survival Trust nurture such animals and help prevent them from disappearing for good.

Then it's on to the pigs, amongst many others to see the unmistakable Gloucester Old Spots and the russet-coloured Tamworths. Then off to the goats, and of course, no trip was complete without going to see all the magnificent latest tractors and farm machinery; the life-size versions, and dare I say much more modern versions, of the farm toys I used to play with as a child.

Later in the afternoon, it was over to see the horses, which were always magnificently turned out. I also got to watch some of my friends compete in the show jumping, which in days gone by was regularly shown on mainstream television but sadly seems more of a niche interest now as far as TV is concerned.

And even now, when I'm close to drawing my pension, I still love that same routine and feel childhood wonder at every show. Over the years, the show has diversified greatly to attract a bigger and wider audience. It is with a tinge of sadness that I feel too many of the public these days are increasingly detached from where their food originates and how it is produced. The stalls selling superb

Yorkshire, through and through

local produce have expanded, the machinery has become bigger and more advanced, and many country crafts and pursuits have been introduced to add to the show's appeal.

There's a real buzz all around the place that visitors and exhibitors can't help but get caught up in. Thanks to the television series *Today at the Great Yorkshire Show*, which I've appeared on for several years, I've been able to get to know the people behind the scenes at the event, and have also followed clients as they prepare for the show when filming *The Yorkshire Vet*. These people run the show with fantastic efficiency and, in true Yorkshire fashion, with a smile on their faces. They are modest people who personify every positive aspect of the Yorkshire character. I feel it is befitting that such people organise what is the country's most prestigious agricultural show.

It's easy to forget when you're there that years and sometimes decades of preparation have gone into developing these show animals to get them to a stage where they're good enough to compete in such a respected event. They are the best in the UK. When it comes to judging, it is incredibly difficult because the animals are so good that, to coin an old-fashioned phrase, you would struggle to put a cigarette paper between them. I had experience of this in 2022 when I was given the opportunity to have a go at judging in one of the show rings while filming *Today at the Great Yorkshire Show*. I was asked to accompany the judge during the Shorthorn bull category, and met a chap called Richard who explained the criteria I should be looking for, and who also made it quite clear from the show committee's perspective that my opinion would be for the cameras only and would not have any bearing on the official scoring. I was moved on before Princess Anne arrived in the ring, and despite only being a warm-up act for the main event,

I thoroughly enjoyed the experience. Whether my attempts held any merit is debatable, as the animals I scored most highly were at the lower end of Richard's scorecard. A few weeks later, my top choice went for official grading and apparently got a grade of 95 per cent, which was very high. That made me feel a lot better. And it was particularly relevant as 2022 marked the 200th anniversary of the establishment of the Beef Shorthorn Cattle Society. In 1822 George Coates published the first volume of his herd book, which was the first pedigree herd book for cattle in the world. It was based on information collected by Coates as he travelled around farms in County Durham on his bike. The data he collected from the stock he visited was used to improve the developing cattle by selecting the better ones to breed from. Really when you think about it, and looking at the animals on display nowadays, this hasn't changed apart from now there is no gentleman going from farm to farm on a push bike collecting information about superior progeny!

Over the years I've watched clients prepare their stock for the show, characters such as Graham Hunt, who farms just outside Thirsk and was originally keeping Dexters before moving to Shorthorns. Graham is a typical County Durham lad, a no-nonsense, no-frills man who knows his stock inside out. He calls a spade a spade and is one of the nicest men you'll ever meet. He's had quite an incredible rise in the breed because in the first year that he showed at the Great Yorkshire Show he got a first prize for one of his bulls and one of his cows. He is a true stockman with an eye for a superior cow or bull. I suppose just like Coates 200 years ago.

Indeed, to win a class is a real plaudit. Farmers will sit up and take notice of a winning bull and acclaimed official recognition is obviously highly prestigious and enhances the value of the stock. Consequently, early in the morning on the day of the show, the

Yorkshire, through and through

farmers and stock handlers will meticulously prepare their animals for showing. The amount of work and titillatiion that goes into getting them show-ready is phenomenal. There's massaging, power-washing, and blow-drying involved. And with some of the sheep, the fleece is dyed as well. As the judging time nears you can cut the tension with a knife.

Then, as the day goes on, and the judging is over, everybody becomes a little more relaxed, and the beers start to flow. The camaraderie is wonderful and there's a lot of laughter, friendship and genuine respect for each other on display. The farmers set up bales and tables between the rows of livestock, and as the afternoon progresses you have cows on one side and cows on the other, with increasingly inebriated farmers in the middle.

Some people will travel if not to the ends of the Earth, to the ends of the UK to find the perfect show animal. A few years ago, I accompanied Rob and Dave Nicholson from Cannon Hall Farm, and their father, Roger, to Oban in Scotland on a mission to buy a Highland cow or heifer for the farm. Again, the idea was to select the best ones available to take home with a view to future showing and breeding, and where else would a Yorkshireman love to compete other than at The Great Yorkshire Show?

The previous evening Lin and I had been at a charity function in London, hosted by Gloria Hunniford to raise funds for the charity set up in her daughter, Caron Keating's, memory. Caron sadly died of cancer in 2004 aged just forty-one. We left the function and flew up to Glasgow, from where we drove to Oban and the Oban Auction Mart, where we saw an absolute beaut of a Highland heifer named Fern.

Obviously, farmers always want to pay as little as possible, and I was with Roger at one side of the collecting ring where the auction was being conducted, while Rob and Dave were on the other side. Fern entered the ring and the bidding started. Bidding at these auctions is done with imperceptible finger-raises or the twitch of an eyelid. Roger began bidding but the higher the price went, the slower his finger went up. Eventually that finger just wouldn't move at all. The trip was being filmed for the Cannon Hall Farm television show *Springtime on the Farm* and there was an expectation, having travelled all that way, that the Nicholsons would be returning with a potential prize cow or heifer.

When Roger stopped bidding, I looked over and saw the anguished, imploring looks of his sons opposite, who were trying to encourage their father to continue bidding. Roger's finger just wouldn't rise and I felt jolted into action.

'Roger, you've got to bid,' I whispered urgently. Roger looked at me with a resigned look in his eye. Slowly and reluctantly his finger rose again, and the gavel went down at £3,200. Ultimately, back at Cannon Hall Farm, Fern had a calf called Ted. Fern was shown at the Great Yorkshire Show in 2019, where she won the coveted red rosette, a first. She is a superb specimen of a Highland cow and wouldn't look out of place on any catwalk. Ted was shown at the Yorkshire Show in 2022 and he got a third prize, so in the end it was worth it. And we still laugh about Roger and his reluctant finger. It 'were typical Yorkshire were that', as might be said. This sentiment encapsulates the dryness of the humour and our propensity to take the mickey out of ourselves and each other. Sometimes we don't see how funny events are until they've happened. Even Roger eventually laughed about it, after he'd written the cheque out and set off back to Yorkshire.

13

Green energy

It was a Sunday, just before midday, and the delicious smell of roasting lamb filled the house. I was thoroughly enjoying my day off. I'd already polished off several cups of tea and a light breakfast of toast earlier, to leave room for Sunday dinner. The day was mapped out. After dinner I planned to collapse on the sofa and watch some telly. Perhaps later I'd go for a walk. I had nothing better to do than eat and relax.

And then the phone rang, and I saw Mrs Green's number appear on the handset. This was not unusual. I spoke to Jeanie most days and saw her and her husband Stephen several times a week when she'd usually ply me with homemade cake, pork pies, pasties from the Sunday Market and a handful of sweets. It was always a pleasure, and often an adventure. If you've seen *The Yorkshire Vet*, you'll know what I mean. Mr and Mrs Green are a force of nature.

I answered, smiling.

'Hello, Mrs Green. What can I do for you this fine Sunday?' I chirped.

Mrs Green, it appeared, was not in the same fine mood as I was.

'Monty's got a lamb 'ere wi' a broken leg. Can you come and fix it? I won't be 'ere. We're going out.' she said abruptly.

I've always found it hard to say no to the Greens. Truth be told, the relationship I have with them goes way beyond a vet-client relationship. They are close friends and I'd known them long before I returned to Thirsk as a practising vet. They were two of my very first clients and have always been loyal and supportive. We have also always indulged in a lot of banter. The lamb in the oven would have to wait. The lamb at the Greens was more important.

'I'll be there as soon as I can,' I said to Jean. The phone clicked and the line went dead. Jean wasn't ever one for polite small talk, but even by her standards I could tell she was not in the best of moods.

The Monty she was talking about was a local chap who kept two pet sheep on her land for grazing. That morning one of them had produced a large lamb.

I explained to Lin that I had some urgent business to attend to and that, all things being well, I should still be back in time for lunch, then I packed my plaster of Paris and drove down to Thirsk and the Green's farm.

Monty was sitting at the picnic table they have in their front yard with the little lamb perched lovingly on his lap.

Monty, who was a down-to-earth character, looked apologetic.

'I found her like this. I haven't a clue how it happened,' he said. It was highly likely that before the lamb could stand after birth he had been inadvertently trodden on by his grossly overweight mother.

The lamb was obviously in discomfort but was being very brave, and only bleated occasionally. I felt the break, which was on the lower front limb, and realised with some relief that it was a dead-easy one to fix.

Green energy

'I need a drop of warm water for the plaster of Paris,' I said to Monty.

'It's okay,' he replied, 'Jean left the kitchen door open when she left.'

I went into the house to get some water. The kitchen was in its usual lived-in state with cats lazing on various bits of furniture and surfaces. There were plates of what looked like stew, which had been abandoned, which puzzled me.

I filled a bowl with water and went back out to set a cast on the limb.

I worked away, applying a cast while Monty gently held the leg forward in place.

'Mrs Green didn't sound too happy today,' I said to Monty.

'No, she's not. She's absolutely livid with Sarah,' he told me. Sarah, who is the couple's only daughter, is also a bit of a character. It is fair to say that, as in many relationships between mothers and teenage daughters, things between Jean and Sarah sometimes got a little strained.

'What's she done now?' I asked.

Monty explained.

'Well, they were going to have stew for their dinner and Sarah thought she would intervene and tipped a whole two-pound bag of sugar into it. Stephen took one mouthful and spat it out. Jean didn't realise at that point that it was full of sugar, so she gave Stephen a mouthful for spitting out her food. Then she tested it herself and realised what had happened. The air was blue, I can tell you. Anyway, now they've all gone down to the White Horse Cafe for fish and chips for their Sunday dinner because the stew was beyond redemption.'

I was laughing away by the time he finished recounting the events, picturing what happened in my mind, complete with Jean's expletives.

I finished applying the cast to the lamb and waited for the plaster to set before packing up my stuff. Monty told me about the sad demise of a mutual acquaintance of ours, which finished the conversation on a solemn note.

I went to throw my non-clinical rubbish away in one of the dustbins at Jean's back door. It was an old-fashioned galvanised type and, surprisingly for those days, it had a black bin liner inside. As I lifted the lid off and peered into the depths of the bin, there was only one item inside. It was a dead hen. I shook my head, bemused and with disbelief. Why on Earth was there a dead hen in the Greens' dustbin?

And that whole episode summed up the Greens to me. You never knew what to expect, but whatever happened was generally unintentionally funny, and sometimes quite bizarre.

You can never be sure what you'll encounter when you visit the Greens. Jean has a home full of cats, some of which live in the house, while others live in the farm buildings. Some of them choose whether to be inside or out on a daily basis. She also has a lurcher-type dog, Reuben, who lives on the sofa, which he is quite happy to share with a few cats. They all get on like one big happy family. Jean loves her cats, and she picks them up and stretches them out and they let her. It's as if she's bewitched them; she can pull them about, and they appear completely oblivious, without a care in the world.

The couple don't have much, and they don't want much. They are not in the least materialistic, but they are incredibly content, and at times they're like two lovestruck teenagers laughing and giggling together. There's something to be learned from the simplistic life they lead in this hectic day and age. They don't have much money, but by God, they're some of the happiest people I know.

Green energy

They married in 1978. The story goes that Jeanie wanted some eggs and she went across the field to Stephen's farm to get some, as she knew he kept hens. They got talking. Stephen lived on his own, his parents having long since passed. By all accounts and by his own admission he wasn't much of a cook, so Jean agreed to cook him some scrambled eggs. They must have been good because within ten days they were engaged and within three months they were married. It really was a whirlwind romance and true love.

A few years ago, the Greens gave up their dairy cows because Stephen was in his late eighties and they were proving a bit of a handful. He had to go into hospital to have a hernia repaired, and the consultant suggested that cows were becoming too much for him. It broke their hearts to sell them off at auction and they went with them to make sure the cows went to good homes, which they did. This sad episode in their lives was filmed and shown on *The Yorkshire Vet*. It was so poignant. Not many people who watched and didn't shed a tear. With close to two million viewers, that was a lot of tears.

Jean's approach to husbandry was always unconventional. They loved their cows like they were their children, and they all had names. There was Peanut, Rachel, Spider, Long Legs and Giraffe, who she used to feed bananas. Jean gave her one last banana at the auction, just before she was sold.

I started looking after their cows when I returned to Thirsk as a young vet in 1982. It was always an experience.

The animals had to be tested for TB at regular intervals and records needed to be up to date and details had to be sent to the Ministry of Agriculture, Fisheries and Food (MAFF). In line with a lot of other Yorkshire farmers, Stephen's record-keeping left a bit to be desired. Getting basic information about ages and ear-tag numbers would often prove to be a challenge.

I'd be in the cow house with Stephen getting ready to test the cows. Farmers would often be on tenterhooks at this stage, hoping their cows would pass the test.

'How old is this one, Steve?' I'd ask.

He'd frown, take his hat off and scratch his head.

'Well, I can't really say. I'm not sure,' he'd say.

'Well, roughly how old is she, Stephen? It doesn't have to be to the month.'

He'd scratch his head some more, as if the motion would dislodge the information from deep inside his brain.

'Well. . . she could be five.'

I'd write '5' in the book and move on to the next cow.

'—but she's had four calves already, so she's got to be a year or two older than that,' Stephen would recall.

I'd scribble out 5, write 7, and move on.

'Do you know, that's her heifer that we're milking at t'other end of cow house, so she's got to be nine if she's a day,' Stephen would say.

And this was how it went on with all the cows.

If you didn't know the Greens and their ways, you might find it frustrating, but it made me laugh and endeared me to them even more.

Calving with the Greens was also an adventure. Occasionally the calves would be a bit big to be born unaided and I'd have to attend to help. I'd use ropes attached to the calf's limbs inside its mother that would allow me to gently ease the calf out. On one occasion, I must have been subconsciously groaning with the exertion because suddenly Sarah appeared behind me, grabbed me around the waist and start pulling me backwards. And then Jean must have thought she could help too and she grabbed Sarah and started pulling as well. It was like a tug o' war team, doing no good whatsoever but showing plenty of enthusiasm. It was a

Green energy

comical sight for anybody watching.

It was at this point that Jean came out with one of her one-liners.

'You do the groaning, son, and we'll do the pulling,' she said.

I did have to be careful, however, and treat Jean's cows with great respect because for some reason that I could never work out, they could all kick out ferociously.

One day I was there treating Spider for mastitis, and just as I went to her rear end to insert my thermometer into the rectum to take her temperature, Jean was starting to warn me that she was a kicker, just as the cow lashed out with her left hind foot and caught me square in the belly. She could kick higher than any one of the most supple of dancers witnessed on 'Strictly Come Dancing'. Spider sent me sprawling backwards, crashing into the wall behind. I lay there in a heap momentarily, struggling to get my breath back.

Jeanie was horrified and her reaction was just typical. The air turned blue. 'Effing cow!' she yelled as she helped me back to my feet.

From that day on, Stephen used a well-known, tried-and-tested technique to distract the cows. This involved holding the cow by the nostrils using the thumb and forefinger before inserting a tong-like set of pliers into the nostrils to help restrain a trying patient. If the udder needed to be examined, Stephen would be restraining our patient with his pliers at the head end whilst Jeanie would hold the tail up vertically, which is another tried-and-tested technique to prevent kicking. It was always a team effort. Anyone witnessing it who was not familiar with such methods would have found it somewhat bizarre.

Sarah recently rang the practice at midnight just before Halloween to say that her dog Reuben must have a toothache because he was quite distressed. The poor lass who was on duty that night had already been out at 11pm, and was woken by Sarah at midnight before having to perform an emergency caesarean on a bitch at 2am. She asked Sarah to keep an eye on the dog and let her know how he was in the morning. We heard nothing the next day, but Sarah called again the following night at midnight.

'I'm just ringing to say that Reuben didn't have a toothache. I've solved the problem,' she explained to the same vet who was on duty again. 'We'd been watching television together, and while watching it, this ghost walked through the room and went through the wall. And that's what upset Reuben.'

Jean has always made a big thing about my birthdays, and for my fiftieth she invited me to her house for afternoon tea. She made a fruit cake and asked a local lady named Betty Price, who is a baking expert, to ice it and put a picture of a boxer dog on it. Jean knew I loved the breed. Betty, however, reported back that she couldn't do boxers, but she could do Dobermans. So, Jean said, 'Okay, put a Doberman on it.' Sarah had also won a bottle of Moet et Chandon Champagne at the fair that year, which she also planned to open for my birthday tea.

I arrived and the table was laid with various nibbles and crisps. The champagne flutes were also out.

Sarah was becoming agitated because she couldn't wait for the cake, and from somewhere in the back of the house screamed: 'Mum, I'm hungry, what can I eat? I can't wait.'

Jean told her to find something to eat.

'Mum, is there anything in the freezer?' she yelled back. It was quite common for mother and daughter to communicate by screaming at each other from one end of the house to the other.

'Yes. Get something out of the freezer,' shouted Jean.

From somewhere in the distance, I heard rummaging and then a microwave being turned on.

Green energy

Jean then presented me with the cake. It was beautifully iced on top of thick marzipan, onto which had been stuck not a photograph of a Doberman, but that of a Rottweiler, cut from a magazine.

'Do you like it?' asked Jean.

'It's lovely,' I said. 'You've gone to so much effort. You really have a heart of gold.'

At that point there was a ping from next door, the sound of some more crashing around through drawers, and Sarah emerged with a lasagne in a bowl that was bubbling like lava, which she plonked down on the table.

Just as we prepared to cut the cake, there was a knock on the door and in walked a local lady named Annie Bargate, who was another great character and looked as though she'd been working out in the fields. Annie could often be seen collecting dandelions for her rabbits from the side of the main road into Thirsk or pushing a pram filled with items of scrap she'd acquired from the hedgebacks on her travels. She too joined in with my fiftieth birthday celebrations.

The whole thing was joyously chaotic and utterly mesmerising.

Now, the Greens loved their cows, and their cats, and Reuben, but of all the animals they kept, their donkeys have held a special place in their hearts, particularly for Stephen, for whom the sight of a donkey brings back fond memories of donkey rides at the seaside when he was a young boy growing up in Whitby. The family have kept several donkeys over the years as pets. Horace was a favourite and lived with them for many years. Horace was what you would call a 'Marmite' character, meaning that you either loved him or you didn't. He was belligerent, he was awkward and he went out of his way to be difficult. But that was just in his nature and the Greens loved him. Generally, donkeys should be kept in pairs because they are social animals who bond closely with each other.

Horace was the exception to this rule. He lived on his own and he was happier that way. He was a grumpy and cantankerous donkey and the Greens tried to introduce him to other companions over the years, but he wasn't having any of it.

Whilst I had a soft spot for Horace, he made no bones about the fact that he hated me. Whenever I was called out to see him, he would be tied up inside a stable and would manage to muscle me up against the wall where he'd try and squeeze the life out of me. He knew exactly what he was doing. He never kicked, he just tried to intimidate. In one early episode of *The Yorkshire Vet*, I treated him for a skin infection. Antibiotics by mouth were not an option for his particular type of problem, so we decided a bath would be curative. Knowing what a cantankerous beast he could be, I took our head nurse, Rachel, for backup, and Steve and Jean were on hand to help too. As usual, Horace tried to crush me against the fence to which he was tied, so I gave him a little bit of a sedative to get him to stand still. It worked well and we managed to give him his bath, which was quite an experience, not only for Horace, but for me as well because it was the first time I'd ever bathed a donkey.

Horace's death was a sad affair. His field backed on to a housing estate and people often walked past and said hello. Mainly, he'd ignore them but if they had treats, he was more inclined to give them the time of day. But this can be very problematic for donkeys because people unknowingly give them food they shouldn't eat. Grass clippings are a classic example. They ferment and produce gas and cause colic. As do fruit and vegetables. Many was the time Jean remonstrated with well-meaning people from the adjacent houses who had almost killed Horace with kindness. Horace was fed a whole lot of food that he shouldn't have had. It sat in his stomach fermenting away, which caused severe colic and a twisted gut and sadly he had to be put to sleep. The Greens were heartbroken and missed having a donkey around and so the call went out to find them a replacement for Horace.

That is how they ended up with Mabel and Sybil, two rescue donkeys who were very fond of each other. Mabel was quite a lot older than Sybil, however, and her health deteriorated relatively quickly. Towards the end she was going off her legs and had no quality of life, so sadly it was kinder to let her go, and she was put to sleep. That left Sybil on her own. Whenever I saw her after that, she always looked thoroughly miserable, standing out there in her paddock, uninterested in life without her best friend to keep her company. She was pining, and although she was still eating, you could tell that inside she was lost, and she just needed a companion. Once again, the challenge was set to find the Greens another donkey, and Sybil a new friend.

One day I was talking to the Nicholson brothers from Cannon Hall Farm and mentioned my quest to find a donkey for the Greens. To my delight they said that they had a youngster for whom they were looking for a good home. His name was Donkey Oti (Don Quixote), and he was just six months old.

There was quite an age gap between Don and Sybil, who was around ten years old, but I hoped having a young upstart around would give the older donkey a new lease of life.

Rob and Dave Nicholson delivered Donkey Oti to the Greens' farm and Jean and Stephen were delighted, although Jean declared straight away that she didn't like that name.

'We're going to call him Fernando,' she declared.

It was a beautiful moment when we introduced the donkeys. Sybil took one look at Fernando, and it was like love at first sight. And from being totally miserable, she brightened up immediately with her new handsome donkey companion. It put the spring back in her step and she looked as if she had a smile on her face. She had a reason to live again, and it brought it home to me very succinctly how donkeys have to be in pairs or groups for companionship in order to live a happy, fulfilled life.

Initially we had to be careful just in case the initial excitement wore off and the donkeys decided that they weren't keen on each other after all. So, for the first few days they were kept in separate calf pens with walls low enough so that they could see each other. This gave them a chance to familiarise themselves with one another, but Fernando was such a loveable character, there was never a chance that they wouldn't get on famously.

Initially Jean told me that she was worried Fernando might get up to some 'funny business' with his new companion. To others, however, she seemed quite excited by the idea that there might be the chance of a donkey foal on the farm. Nevertheless, when I checked Fernando, it transpired that only one of his testicles had descended. We waited until both were fully descended and then he was castrated. I performed the procedure with the help of the very capable and professional Shona Searson, a brilliant vet who works at Donaldson's, the practice in Huddersfield who look after Cannon Hall Farm and also appear on *The Yorkshire Vet*.

'Fernando's from your part of the world; it'll be nice for him to have somebody from South Yorkshire that speaks the lingo,' I joked, knowing that Fernando was technically from South Yorkshire, whereas the Donaldson's practice is in West Yorkshire

When Fernando and Sybil were finally let free together in the field, it was a joy to behold. Sybil was like a teenager again, rolling around in the grass in pure delight. They got along famously from that day on and are inseparable. The Greens love them both, knowing that Fernando and Sybil have the perfect life there.

14

Donkeys, ducks and wildlife

Anyone who knows donkeys will understand why the Greens have such a bond with theirs. You can't help but love them, with their dour expressions and stoic fortitude. How can you not love donkeys? You look at the face of a donkey and there's something comforting about it, and, if I dare say so, their oversized ears look a little bit comical, which adds to their charm.

Anyone who is old enough to have had donkey rides as a youngster will most likely have a special affinity with them. Some of my fondest childhood memories are of donkey rides on the beach at Scarborough. My granny used to take my brother and me and we'd sit there atop a donkey each as they plodded along serenely. There was never any suggestion that they were going to run off. It felt totally secure and I loved it. They always looked so docile and approachable, standing there in a little group on the sand, letting the passers-by pat them and then plodding across the beach with children on their backs. They took everything in their stride and at their own pace.

I was used to horses, so found it fascinating that donkeys ate from nosebags, not from troughs. That tickled me as a youngster, watching them snacking on the beach, on their well-earned lunchbreak.

The rides on the beach were the first significant contact I had with donkeys, and then, when I qualified as a vet, I started to treat them, because there was always somebody who had a donkey or a couple of donkeys on their land. Although they appear as quite hardy animals, donkeys, I discovered, do not have as much protective oil in their coats as horses and ponies, so they are far more susceptible to the wet. For this reason, it is important that they have somewhere to shelter when the weather turns wet and miserable. It's also important that they have a hard-standing because their hooves, which are not particularly robust, will soften if they are continually wading in mud. Like horses and ponies, they also need a dental technician to look at them regularly and make sure their teeth are okay.

I also started to discover that because they are such docile, unobsrusive animals, there is a tendency for them to be abused and neglected. Even some of those beach donkeys, which I always assumed as a boy were happy and well looked after, were not being cared for as much as they should have been, much to my dismay.

In 2018, I took part in a Channel Five telethon called *Help the Animals*, which several animal charities benefited from, one of which was The Donkey Sanctuary, the biggest equine charity in the world. As part of the event, I was asked to travel down to The Donkey Sanctuary's headquarters in Devon to make a short film about the charity's work, which was to be shown on the night. I learned that they had 7,000 donkeys under their care and ran state-of-the-art operating facilities with a laboratory and a team of vets, nurses and people trained to look after donkeys and help them back to full health. The donkeys in their care live in a beautiful setting with acres of grazing space. They end up at The Donkey Sanctuary for several different reasons. Some have been neglected or abused. Some have been abandoned. Some have been pets that their owners could no longer look after, perhaps because of old age or death, or because of a marriage split where the property and land had to be sold. The charity also runs a network of welfare officers all over the country, who offer free advice to donkey owners.

Well, when we filmed the clip for the telethon, I fell in love with the place. If anyone is feeling a bit down in the dumps, a trip to The Donkey Sanctuary cannot fail to lift their spirits. I came out of there floating on air. One of the most heart-warming sights happened in the morning when the donkeys were let out from their overnight accommodation. The huge yard doors were thrown open and all these braying donkeys came belting out into the sunshine. It was a joy to behold, particularly as many of them that had been abused or neglected were restored to full physical and psychological health.

While I was there, I also helped one of the vets remove a large malignant sarcoid from a resident donkey called Poppy. I was wowed by just how mindful of the needs of the donkeys the staff were. Like most of the donkeys there, the patient had been paired with a mate and they were inseparable. We walked Poppy and her best friend Delilah down to the theatre together and Delilah stayed in a special pen next to the theatre while Poppy had the surgery. And as soon as she came round and was sufficiently recovered, she was taken to be with her mate again.

The Donkey Sanctuary is also very much an international organisation, and a large part of their remit is to improve the lives of donkeys in countries where they are still used as beasts of burden, and where remote communities in Africa and Asia, particularly, rely on them to carry clean water and other loads. These communities can't function very well without their donkeys. These lovely animals do so much good in this world, and so to abuse and neglect them is unforgivable.

The Donkey Sanctuary works with various African communities to educate them on donkey health and welfare and to provide medical assistance when needed. It also raises the profile and status of the donkey through numerous thoughtful initiatives and diplomacy.

At the telethon event in the Leeds TV studios, I met Dawn, the granddaughter of the charity's founder, Dr Elisabeth Svendsen, a Yorkshire woman who knew how to get things done. Dawn knew how much I'd enjoyed my visit and asked me if I'd consider becoming the ambassador for the charity, as the following year was the fiftieth anniversary of its foundation and they'd never had an ambassador before. I was honoured and jumped at the chance to be part of such a wonderful organisation that through kind public donations makes a huge difference to the wellbeing of donkeys worldwide.

One of the other major issues affecting the global donkey population in the past few years has been the horrific trade in donkeys in order to fuel a demand for a compound found in donkey skin that is used in Traditional Chinese Medicine (TCM). The substance, called ejiao, is a gelatinous glue-like substance created by boiling donkey skin. It is believed to have a range of health benefits.

The supply of donkeys has pretty much been exhausted in China, and there continues to be such a demand that prices have been driven high enough to make it worthwhile for unscrupulous donkey traders to steal donkeys from communities at gunpoint and slaughter them for their skins.

The Donkey Sanctuary has investigated this trade for several years, and the figures and details they have uncovered are shocking. For example, in 2016 it was estimated that 5,600 tonnes of ejiao were produced, requiring 4.8 million donkey skins. The China-based industry sourced approximately 1.8 million of these skins domestically. The remaining three million were sourced through a largely unreported global donkey skin trade. The number could have been much higher, as a spokesperson for one of China's biggest ejiao producers, Dong-E-E-Jiao, confirmed that China imported 3.5 million donkey skins in 2016. As investigators dug deeper, they discovered a vast international network of donkey traders – some of whom were legal and authorised, whilst others were illegal and linked to organised crime, involving the use of marauding gangs of heavily armed thieves to steal donkeys from impoverished communities.

China's domestic donkey herd has rapidly depleted. Chinese agricultural authorities reported that donkey numbers reduced from an estimated 11 million in 1990 to around six million in 2014. Present estimates suggest there are only around two million donkeys left in China.

In January 2017, The Donkey Sanctuary published *Under the Skin*, its first ground-breaking report into this appalling trade. The report foreword described how villagers in one rural community in Tanzania woke one morning to find all their twenty-four hard-working donkeys had been stolen, killed, and stripped of their skins overnight. In 2022 the Tanzanian government closed a slaughterhouse for donkeys, where officials found 800 of these poor creatures waiting to be slaughtered, many of which had been stolen from local communities. The Donkey Sanctuary were instrumental in rehoming these donkeys and helping make their accommodation secure enough to ensure that they couldn't be easily stolen again.

The charity's work exposing this barbarity continues, as does its work in other parts of the world. Indeed, the year before the pandemic I planned a trip to Nepal and East India with The

Donkey Sanctuary to film a documentary showing its work in clinics there treating injured and ill donkeys, particularly those used in the brick-making industry. The documentary was due to be shown on *The Yorkshire Vet*, but unfortunately, Covid put a stop to the plans.

More recently, I was asked to help make a small film celebrating the fifth anniversary of the charity's new operating facilities, located at Brookfield Farm in Devon. These facilities are not open to the public, so the film allowed a behind-the-scenes look. Between opening in 2017 and when I visited in 2022, over 1,500 donkeys had been operated on there. The site also carries out research into conditions that donkeys are prone to suffer from. One such condition is called keratoma, which is a benign tumour of the inner layers of the hoof wall. The contrast of the facilities there and the conditions I sometimes had to work in out in the field were stark. There was no such thing as administering an anaesthetic and then chasing a half-sedated animal around a field, as I sometimes had to do. Everything at The Donkey Sanctuary hospital was designed to make the process as stress-free as possible for the patient. . . And for the veterinary surgeon.

On the day I visited, the patient was a donkey called Dopey, who was part of a group of seven who were all named after the Seven Dwarves. Dopey needed an operation because he had a sarcoid growing on his preputial sheath. There are different ways of treating the condition. One method is to restrict the blood flow to the growth by using an elasticated ligature placed around the base of the tumour. The growth then dies and drops off. There is also a cream that can be used. It is called 'Liverpool Cream' and was developed by a professor at Liverpool University Veterinary School. It is highly toxic and can only be applied by vets. These growths cannot be removed by conventional surgery with a scalpel because they tend to quickly grow back at the original site. The gold standard modern treatment is to laser the sarcoid off. Laser treatment has been shown to be the most effective method of stopping regrowth at the original site of the tumour.

To keep Dopey's stress levels to a minimum he was walked to just outside the operating theatre with his mate Doc and then taken inside and given a check over to make sure he was fit and well for the surgery. He was given pre-op sedatives and then walked through to an area called the 'knockdown box', which was next door to the theatre and not as bad as it sounds. It is a lovely, comfortable, heated and padded area in which the induction anaesthetic is administered. Once Dopey was asleep, having collapsed on the comfortable padded floor, a large winch attached to the ceiling on rails was manoeuvred over him, and hobbles (straps for the legs), which were connected to the winch, were attached to his lower limbs. He was then slowly lifted by the winch and the conveyor system took him through to the operating room, where he was lowered down onto the operating table. An endotracheal tube was inserted into his windpipe to administer a maintenance anaesthetic, the levels of which were closely monitored by one of several nurses assisting in the procedure. All vets and nurses were in sterile protective clothing and had scrubbed up in an area adjacent to the theatre. Everything was done properly, following the same procedures as in a human operating theatre.

Those in attendance wore Crocs that didn't leave the operating site, so as to minimise cross-contamination and any infection risk.

With Dopey stable under the anaesthetic, the vet had as long as was needed to carry out the surgery. They had control of the depth and duration of the anaesthesia by maintaining him on gaseous anaesthetic mixed with oxygen via the tube inserted in his upper airways. This was unlike my experiences in the field, where there is often a rush to finish a procedure before the anaesthetic wears off. This happened to me recently when I was applying some elastic bands to some skin sarcoids on the underside of a horse and the patient got up just before I had finished.

The levels of concentration within the operating theatre were impressive. Everyone knew exactly what was required of them and the atmosphere was one of quiet professionalism. The procedure ran like clockwork. The only thing that mattered in the room was the patient.

Once the white-hot laser had done its work and the procedure was finished, Dopey was lifted back into the knockdown box where he came round whilst being carefully monitored. As soon as he was back on his legs again, he was taken out to where Doc, his best friend, was waiting for him. Samples from the removed masses were sent to the onsite laboratory for analysis. The results showed that the chance of recurrence of these horrible skin tumours was virtually zero. Sadly, even with state-of-the-art surgical procedures, this positive outcome is not always the case, since one of the others in the group, Dopey, suffered the same condition and had to be put to sleep.

It just so happened that seventy-two hours previously, I'd castrated the Greens' donkey, Fernando, and I'd been to see another lovely little donkey called Bertie the same day, who was lame due to an infection in his foot causing an abscess which I pared out and drained. As I watched the high-tech procedure at The Donkey Sanctuary, I couldn't help but marvel at how far advanced the facilities were. Even though I do not have an envious bone in my body, I did think how different my life could have been with such facilities.

I was honoured to help The Donkey Sanctuary and I see it as a great privilege to be their ambassador.

Donkeys, ducks and wildlife

There may be an unfair image sometimes of vets as money-grabbing opportunists, but we all enter this profession because of our love and respect for animals, and we want to help. I've known several colleagues who have gone on to work for conservation organisations. One such person and one of my best friends is Andy Routh, a typical dyed-in-the-wool Yorkshireman who I shared a house with at Liverpool Veterinary School. He works at the world-famous Gerard Durell Conservation Trust on Jersey. Andy has devoted his life to helping endangered species all over the world and I am very proud to call him my friend.

In Thirsk, on a fairly regular basis, when people find injured wild animals, it is quite common for them to bring them into the practice where we will do what we can for them. In fact, one former Kirkgate client even had a pet fox, which she'd hand-reared and walked around town on a leash and collar, and which we spayed and vaccinated.

One such urgent case was rescued from the banks of the Cod Beck, a stream which runs through Thirsk, winding through the middle of the town and then following the path south, down to Topcliffe, where it feeds into the River Swale, which eventually runs into the River Ouse and empties into the Humber Estuary and the North Sea.

Cars trundle over the stream on Bridge Street as they leave the market square, and underneath the bridge, the clear water babbles over the shallows, which are overhung by willow and sycamore trees. It is an idyllic scene, with a footpath running from the bridge along the bank where families walk and often stop to feed the ducks. What could be more serene than feeding the ducks in the spring? Unfortunately for Kevin the duck (who was a female, but I'll explain that later), the Cod Beck was not such a peaceful place.

She was discovered by a young chap and his parents, who had been out walking by the beck side. The other ducks had set upon her, and she was being pecked mercilessly when the family intervened and rescued her. She had sustained several injuries; her head was swollen and bleeding, and you could not see her eyes due to the trauma to her eyelids. She was so weak and exhausted that the boy was able to get hold of her and put her into a box. The family then brought her into the surgery where I examined her.

She looked in a terrible state, but on closer inspection most of the injuries were fairly superficial. *We can do something here*, I thought, *we can probably save her.* I was heartened by this because in my experience, by the time wildlife arrive at the surgery, they are usually too far gone to save. The patients are often too weak, chronically ill or emaciated, or the injuries are so severe that the only option is euthanasia. Around 75 per cent of wildlife cases brought to vets sadly have to be put to sleep.

But Kevin had a chance. And the injuries, although they looked horrific, were treatable. The main problems were her eyes, which were incredibly traumatised and needed to have ointment applied to them every day. Cream also needed to be applied to the head lesions to help them heal and prevent secondary infection. Kevin also needed painkillers.

As I worked on the injuries, the little lad who saved the duck watched with a concerned look.

'Do you have anywhere you could look after her?' I asked.

Kevin would need time to convalesce.

The boy was keen to take the duck back to his house and look after her, but his parents explained that they lived on a housing estate and that they only had a normal garden and no pond, and the neighbours had cats, so it wasn't an ideal environment for a duck. The boy was quite upset. I think he'd had his heart set on nursing the duck back to health.

Donkeys, ducks and wildlife

I thought for a second. My home was in the countryside outside Thirsk; I had a pond and I had space.

'I'll take her home if you like,' I said to the boy. 'I can look after her.'

'Can't he come back with us?' the boy begged his parents, with tears welling in his eyes (he thought the hen was a drake).

'I promise you, I'll look after her,' I said. 'I'll get her better.'

The parents persuaded their son that it was the right thing to do. I decided to gently let the little lad know that his duck was a she.

'What do you call her?' I asked.

'She's called Kevin,' the boy said.

'Kevin?' I repeated.

'Yeah, she's Kevin.' He replied defiantly.

So, Kevin the duck made a journey home with me, where I set up a shelter for her. I had a cloche in the garden that I used to keep butterflies off my vegetables, and I placed half of it on the lawn and half of it across the pond. I placed a large cardboard box filled with bedding under the mesh-covered cloche, so she had warmth and shelter from predators. She settled in fine, was safe and had access to the pond. Each morning and night I put ointment in her eyes and smeared antiseptic cream over her head. Gradually she recovered. The feathers started to grow back. The injuries healed and Kevin seemed quite content, quacking around the lawn or bobbing happily on the water within the confines of my garden cloche.

One morning I got up and went out to check on her. She had disappeared from under the cloche. Initially I was worried that a fox had taken her in the night, but I looked everywhere and there were no feathers, which you usually find when a fox has attacked. Kevin had been quite strong at this point and had been doing very nicely. In the woods opposite, there were some duck ponds, so I was as certain as I could be that Kevin had done a runner. She'd released herself.

Up until that point we had never seen a duck on our pond, or on our land for that matter, but the following year I woke one morning, looked out of the window to the garden and there on the pond were a duck and a drake, quite happily swimming around. The duck had a slightly bald head. I'm sure as I can be that it was Kevin and her boyfriend. Ducks do return to places they know, and we've never had any other ducks there prior to Kevin or since. They stayed there all day but were gone by the time I returned home from work. Nevertheless, I was absolutely chuffed to know that Kevin was fine, fully recovered and had found herself a true mate.

One of the greatest pleasures I get in life is seeing the wildlife in and around my home, and we are lucky enough to live opposite some beautiful woodland where several barn owls hunt at night. They are shy and elusive creatures, but it always thrills me when I see one swooping out of the woods and into the open, over the house. They are the most graceful creatures that you could possibly imagine. They are silent and designed in such a way as to make them superb hunters. They have incredible sight and hearing that is so acute they can hear a mouse or a vole running in the grass from a vast distance away. Their head is designed in such a way as to direct sound to their ears. They have dampers on their feathers, so they fly virtually silently. When they swoop in and pounce, the force of the strike on their prey is the equivalent of a human being hit by a double-decker bus. The quarry dies instantly.

I'll never forget the thrill of seeing a barn owl hunting at dusk the first winter we moved to our present home in 2006. Each night he'd emerge and silently and almost ghostlike he would fly past the front, looking for food. I'd wait for him and watch in amazement. But it was a hard winter and eventually his nightly forays stopped.

Donkeys, ducks and wildlife

Most likely, he couldn't find enough food and couldn't survive. For that reason, I started to put food out to help any owls in the vicinity. Other owls soon arrived at the owl box that had a protruding platform on which the food was placed. It's become a regular part of my routine now, and the woods come alive at night with the noise of owls hooting and screeching. It's not just barn owls that help themselves to the food on offer at the Wright owl buffet, we get tawny and little owls too. Sometimes they perch on the weathervane on top of the shed waiting for me to go and feed them. They won't come down when I'm visible, but sometimes if I go and hide behind the greenhouse, I'll see these beautiful creatures swoop down and grab the food. It's just a fleeting moment but it gives me so much pleasure watching them.

I always hoped one of the females would nest in my owl box but they never have. However, a farmer friend of mine, Maurice, who lives half a mile away across the fields as the crow flies, also feeds the owls and has several boxes in strategic places on his land too. He rang one Saturday morning, his voice quaking with emotion because of his five boxes, three of them had pigeons in them, one was empty, and that morning in the fifth box he discovered several white bundles of fluffy feathers; one of the barn owls was raising a brood.

'Do you know,' he said, 'if I won £1,000,000 from the lottery, I couldn't be happier.' And the lucky man has had several broods in his boxes since. And it's sometimes said that farmers are hard-hearted!

And Kevin wasn't the only wild visitor I looked after. A while ago, a builder friend was renovating an old building and unwittingly disturbed a hedghog's nest. In it was a mother and five babies.

He called me, quite upset.

'What do I do with these? I can't leave them here on this building site,' he said.

I told him to bring them up to me, and I built them a little house on the grass near my vegetable garden with bricks and a slab of concrete on top as a secure roof. I filled it with hay, and I put it near the vegetable patch because there were lots of slugs and snails there for them to eat. The 'guests' moved in and, although I didn't disturb them and didn't see them because they are nocturnal, I could tell they were happy and going about their business because they left plenty of hedgehog poo about. Eventually the amount of poo started to diminish as the youngsters grew up and moved on, until finally one day there was none.

Folks, quite rightly, love wildlife, and we have plenty of people in and around North Yorkshire who run small rescue centres for such creatures, whose aim is to treat and look after injured or abandoned animals and then return them to the wild. These are not as grand as The Donkey Sanctuary, but they all do their bit to look after the multitude of animals that sometimes just need a bit of human help and kindness.

15

Goodbye Skeldale

The veterinary profession I find myself working in today is almost unrecognisable from the one I stepped into back in 1982 when I returned to Thirsk and to the cosy embrace of Kirkgate, with all its characters and escapades. It is fair to say that I miss those days, but veterinary practice continues to be a rewarding career, and there are still echoes of the old days in some of the places and people I work with.

Veterinary practice has to move with the times, and while I keep abreast of new methods and techniques, I'm not a fool. Admittedly, I am a bit of a dinosaur and one day it will be time for me to hang up my stethoscope.

One of the biggest changes for vets of my generation and in my part of the world has undoubtedly been the dramatic change in farming, which has a knock-on effect for vets who have a large farming clientele.

Back in the Herriot days, the landscape was dotted with lots of small family-owned farms which kept little dairy herds of up to thirty or so cows and a flock of fifty sheep. These farmers were not in it to make big money. It was a way of life passed down through generations. They made a living, but they didn't get rich. As a vet looking after this kind of clientele, life was one light-hearted negotiation after another with farmers who watched every penny and grumbled each time your services were required.

'By 'eck, lad. 'Ow much?' was a common refrain.

As time went by, these small family farms began to disappear. The sons and daughters didn't follow their parents' path and were unwilling to work seven days a week in hard conditions for little recompense. Larger farming enterprises subsequently swallowed these farms up. Food prices continuously declined and supermarkets squeezed the margins so tightly that even now some of the larger farms struggle to make a reasonable living. This has altered the structure of the countryside and the rural economy.

For rural veterinary practices, this has meant that year on year, the number of farming clients and farm animal work has gradually dwindled. When I first started working back in Thirsk, the split between large animal work and small animal work would be roughly 65 per cent farm and large animals and 35 per cent small animals. But even in the 1980s, the trend was moving towards more companion animal work.

Going back twenty years, mixed veterinary practices, such as Kirkgate and Skeldale in its early years, were the backbone of the profession. Now they're considered to be archaic because most practices specialise in one discipline or another, while some farm enterprises are so big that they employ vets in-house, although that hasn't worked out particularly well for the farms I know.

In 1982, Kirkgate looked after between fifty and sixty small dairy herds. When I left Skeldale in 2020, we had one dairy herd left. With fewer, larger farms which were doing more of the work themselves, vets became drug suppliers, supplying antibiotics and vaccines to beef-fattening units, some of which had 1200-plus fattening cattle. A vet would visit maybe once every couple of months or so. Occasionally we were called to dehorn some cattle or carry out numerous pregnancy diagnoses or deal with a pneumonia outbreak.

In this competitive environment, every penny counts, and those that can supply drugs cheaper and buy in bulk gain an advantage. In the old days, geography was important. Local farms employed local veterinary practices. Now there are representatives from big corporate chains based up to forty miles away who have the purchasing power to buy vast quantities of drugs cheaply, roaming the land with price lists, undercutting local veterinary practices and securing contracts with the enterprises. The result is an irate farmer on the phone complaining that a bloke from miles away says he can charge several pence a shot less than you can for a certain drug, so why can't you match him? As a vet from a local community practice, you would sometimes go to a client to see a sick animal and see stocks of drugs in their medicine cabinet from one of the large farm veterinary enterprises, knowing that you had been undercut but unable to do anything about it. It was soul-destroying and it ripped the heart out of community farm and mixed veterinary practices such as Skeldale.

At Skeldale, in order to try and remain competitive in this environment, we ended up supplying one particular respiratory vaccine to one particular farm where we made one penny profit on five doses of vaccine. When I worked that out, I had to ask myself, what's the point? And with margins for veterinary care cut to the bone, is that good for animal welfare? I don't know, but farmers look at the pounds and pence. I have heard that some farm vets are carrying out veterinary services for as little as £40 an hour. If you get your car serviced or you need another trade, you probably pay around £70 to £100 an hour. For a large animal practice, unless you specialise in horse work where the economies are different, it's a financial race to the bottom. The Herriot-type client has all but disappeared around Thirsk. My old boss, Alf Wight, and his son Jim, could see the writing on the wall back in the early nineties. I remember one day the surgery was full of dogs, and they both said to me, 'Peter, this is the future of the veterinary practice.' I didn't quite grasp it at that point but I do now.

Eventually at Skeldale we were almost doing the farm work at a loss. The farm work was being subsidised by the small animal work. I was very aware that towards the end of my time there, I was doing farm work purely for sentimental reasons because I loved doing it, and I loved the characters, but they too were dying out and being replaced by farming enterprises run purely on a business basis, not as a way of life. You can't have banter and a brew with a spreadsheet.

Another effect of this fundamental shift away from mixed veterinary practice has been the difficulty in recruitment. I latterly interviewed many young vets for jobs at Skeldale who asked what percentage of our work is small animals and what is farm? They wanted more farm animal work than we could offer and when they realised we couldn't provide it they went elsewhere, because there was such a shortage of vets they had a massive choice of jobs available.

Veterinary practice has always been seen as a Cinderella profession. Training takes years and it requires a lot of study and dedication. Young people can get a degree now and go and work in the city and earn much larger salaries for much less effort. Compared

Goodbye Skeldale

with accountancy and law we've always been the poor relative. And I can understand why when you look at the hours you've got to work as a vet, particularly if you don't work in a practice where night cover is outsourced. You end up working seven days a week with night cover for an average wage, and for many years now UK practices have looked overseas to fill their vacancies.

The profession has moved and changed at a great pace, and it become harder for young graduates to be able to take in all the requirements, skills and knowledge needed in all species. This then begs the question: Is the veterinary degree fit for purpose? There is so much specialism within the profession now that there is a valid argument for graduates to specialise too, because increasingly the practices they apply to work in will specialise, be that in farm, equine or small animal work, where there is now an even greater degree of specialisation in branches such as orthopaedics, cardiology and medicine, as well as in exotic species mentioned earlier.

Two decades ago, each advertised role would have attracted a few dozen applicants at Skeldale. In 2017, we advertised for an assistant and we received three applicants, one each from Italy, Bulgaria and Pakistan. The Pakistani applicant wanted to be offered a job without an interview because he wasn't going to travel all the way from Pakistan for an interview. Now, when young vets come for an interview, it's almost as if they're interviewing you. They ask about work-life balance, how many nights a week will they be expected to work, or how many weekends a month will they be on call. When they are told they will be working two weekends out of four, they're not interested. Whereas with myself, Jim, and Tim, and an assistant, two of us would work up until a Saturday lunchtime and then we increased up to three because the Saturday morning workload got busier and busier. And from Saturday lunchtime, two of us would be on call for the rest of the weekend. The pattern worked out that we'd have one weekend off in three. If someone was on holiday, we'd work every other night on duty, plus the days, plus the weekend. Graduates in this day and age will rarely put up with that workload. Who can blame them?

I mention all this not because I'm moaning (there are plenty of other professions which have changed beyond all recognition in the past few decades), but to explain why, in 2017, Tim and I decided to sell Skeldale to a corporate organisation. By that stage I had seen the writing on the wall too and understood that as it was, Skeldale just couldn't survive. In business terms, we were stable with an exceedingly good small animal client base and a reasonable balance sheet; however, the issue was staffing. We just couldn't compete for talent because the old ways of working in a mixed species veterinary practice, where you are on call for such long periods, just didn't wash with the new generation of vets graduating from university. Having been absent from so many family milestones myself when I was working, I could fully understand them.

The company we sold to, Medivet, had around 260 practices, and ultimately supplied a dedicated night team for some of its practices, including Thirsk. That meant we could employ vets solely for day work, which allowed us to compete much more favourably in the job market where Millennials didn't want their jobs to be the be-all and end-all of their lives. The company also provided a career structure for vets. They could move between practices. They could specialise in areas such as small animal orthopaedics because the corporate organisations have the infrastructure for them to be able to do so. The wages were also more competitive. New graduates were mentored for three months and didn't have to do any significant work, so they could ease into their working lives gaining confidence in the workplace rather than being thrown in at the deep end. Nurses also were on a much more structured career path.

There were also downsides to the sale of Skeldale to a corporate, but I was convinced it was the only way forward if Skeldale was to thrive in the years to come as the profession continued to change. As part of the sales agreement, I was bound to stay as a partner at Skeldale for two years, which I did. At times I had very heated discussions and arguments with the owners over the way they wanted to run a market town veterinary practice in rural North Yorkshire. It wasn't always easy, and I struggled with some of the working practices that the new owners wanted us to introduce. For example, they wanted us to provide bill estimates to clients so the clients knew how much a treatment was likely to cost before they authorised us to start. I can see how this idea might work in principle, but in reality, it upset a lot of clients. These estimated costs were only ever an indication because often, as a case progressed, more peripheral expenses would be incurred, but it laid claim to the belief that the practice were now only interested in money. Our fees had to go up too, because at the time of the new owners arriving, there was an explosion in vet and nurse salaries as well as the huge costs of running a dedicated night service. Other local independent practices found similar issues, and in order to provide the work-life balance desired by young vets and nurses, they decided not to offer a dedicated night service and are sending clients up to thirty miles away for any out-of-hours or emergency services they may need. Only clients can decide if this type of service is acceptable.

So there were positive benefits, but there were also negatives. However, I knew Skeldale couldn't continue as it was in the challenging and competitive veterinary world we had found ourselves in. The practice might have soldiered on as it was for another few years or so but wouldn't have gone any longer than that. So that's why we made the decision we did, and I stayed there for the required two-year period. When that ended, I had it in my mind that it was going to be closure for me as a veterinary surgeon. It was time to leave, and I was planning to retire.

As my leaving day grew near, I tried to blank it out because it was too much of a fundamental change in my life to comprehend. Skeldale was such a huge and integral part of my life.

Lin always said in our marriage there was her and there was Skeldale. That's how it was. Sadly, sometimes Skeldale came first. I missed the kids growing up. I never went to their nativity plays. I never went to parent-teacher evenings. It sometimes caused conflict because I was never there. Even now I feel guilty because it's time I can't get back. It weighs on my conscience, but I can't turn the clock back, so I've got to move on and accept that's how it was. My problem was, I could never say no. When someone rang and asked specifically for me personally to attend to their animals, it was in my nature to drop everything and go. I can't change what I was, even though sometimes I was dead on my feet.

Walking out of the door of Skeldale for the last time was a huge wrench. There were so many memories, and leaving the staff and the clients, who had become friends, felt like a bereavement. It was very hard, and it was painful. But the time had come for me to move on. It had become more intense, seeing one client after the other at fifteen-minute intervals throughout the day. After so many years, and, dare I say it, as I was getting older, I was getting knackered, and I needed a change of pace.

The funny thing is, when your roots are so far ingrained in a place, you can never really leave. Clients I used to have at Skeldale still ask for me and I still see them around town. Several months after I left, I got a message from Sarah, who is the senior partner there now and doing a fantastic job.

'Did you have a nice holiday?' she said. 'Any problem with travel?'

And then straight to business.

'I had Bramble in today. He's not doing very well. His vision, mobility and breathing are not good. Mrs Wood is not keen to do much with him and is considering euthanasia. I said I will check with you if you would be willing to do it when the time comes, as she misses you and says you've always looked after her dogs.'

This was not an issue for me. I just want to give the support people like Mrs Wood and Bramble need. Sarah said she was happy for me to attend when the time comes because I had known them for so long.

Bramble was a little pug that I'd looked after for years. I was part of his life, and he was part of mine. The type of veterinary work I did at Skeldale was not just a job, it was who I was, and it followed me when I left.

I couldn't say no to Bramble.

16

Hello Grace Lane

When I was nearing the end of my two-year period at Skeldale, I had some big decisions to make. I was at a fork in the road. *The Yorkshire Vet* was still being filmed and was as popular as ever, even after five years. Although the company that made it, Daisybeck, were never sure how long Channel Five would keep commissioning it, they were confident that it wasn't going to be cancelled any time soon. I was soon to be a free agent, and frankly, I was tired, and I was considering packing up altogether.

I went home to Lin one day after work and I had pretty much made up my mind.

'I don't know what to do. I don't know what you think but I'm thinking of retiring,' I told her.

She looked at me in the way she does, with a look of bemusement and concern.

'Well, I don't want you under my feet all day long,' she retorted.

And in that brief exchange my decision was made for me. I was not retiring anytime soon. There were some things to work out, however.

Hello Grace Lane

'But we're no longer doing farm work at Skeldale. I can't change what I am, and I've been a mixed practice vet all my life. I love the small animal work, don't get me wrong, but I don't want to do it all day long, it's too intense.'

Lin listened patiently while I had my moan.

'I want to be able to go out to farms. I want to do some horse-work. I want to continue dealing with lambing difficulties but I also want to continue seeing dogs and cats. I can't change what I've done all my life.'

She nodded along, waited until I'd finished and then said: 'Well, find somewhere else then.'

I thought about that for the next few days, and like the mists on the Moors on a spring morning, my mind began to clear, and I could see a way forward.

My concerns that my traditional veterinary way of life was disappearing had not been completely self-indulgent. The landscape had changed and there wasn't the opportunity for a vet like me to continue working as I had done in Thirsk. But further afield, there were still a few mixed practices working with family-owned farms. One such practice was Grace Lane Vets, which had been set up single-handedly in 2008 by a chap called Stephen Hudson. It was originally located in the middle of the North York Moors in a village called Hutton le Hole and moved to new purpose-built premises in Kirkbymoorside as it grew. In 2013 Stephen was joined by another vet, John Whitwell, who became a partner in the business. The practice did a mix of small animal, farm, and equine work.

I had always admired Grace Lane from afar. It did just the right mix of work that I loved, and I watched the practice grow and develop. They had a great reputation and gave their clients a first-class service. They also invested back into the business and had continued to expand and take on new staff. They had ten vets working there. It was the kind of place I could see myself working and it took me back to when we moved out of 23 Kirkgate to our new premises at Skeldale, which we designed and built over twenty-five years ago.

I contacted Daisybeck (the TV film production company) and explained my plans. I told them I was leaving Skeldale and was considering approaching another practice to see if I could work with them. The team were on board with the plan, and so I contacted John at Grace Lane to sound him out on a proposal.

'This might sound like a strange request,' I began, 'but we're still making *The Yorkshire Vet* and I wondered if you'd be interested in me joining you.'

John didn't have to think for long. I'd like to think his enthusiasm was driven by the opportunity to have me on his team, but it was more likely because as a shrewd businessman he understood the publicity value of being part of such a successful television franchise.

'I'd like to have a chat about that, Peter. That appeals,' he said.

A week or so later, Paul Stead, the chief executive of Daisybeck, Mike Sinclair, the series editor, and I met John Whitwell and Stephen Hudson for a meal at The Pheasant Hotel at Harome. It was a lovely night and John and Stephen were even more delightful than I expected. We discussed how the arrangement might work. At the end of the meal, Mike and Paul left to travel back to Leeds, and John said to me that even if I didn't continue making *The Yorkshire Vet*, he'd like me to work with them, which confirmed to me that I'd made the right decision.

And that's how I ended up with a renewed sense of purpose working with some wonderful colleagues and clients at Grace Lane Vets. While I'm not full-time there, I have the freedom to work as and when I want. I suppose you could say I'm part of the gig economy now. Lin is equally pleased because I'm not under her feet either, so it's a win-win situation.

Grace Lane is a very vibrant practice. There is a lot going on and they cover all aspects of veterinary work. Sadly, I can see they are under the same pressures from the farming practice work as we were at Skeldale, with competition from other vet practices that now maraud all over North Yorkshire, but they are well-equipped to tackle the challenges as they present themselves. They are already extending their premises, and John is always thinking ahead. They are developing a dedicated orthopaedic operating theatre and a laparoscopic spay theatre to add to the two they already have, and are also in the process of building an imaging suite complete with a CT scanner.

John is in his forties and in his prime. He has the knowledge and expertise to take the practice forward. While I'm long in the tooth now, in some ways I'm very like him, but the flesh is weaker these days. It is still very exciting to be part of the story, and Grace Lane's evolution will be shown on *The Yorkshire Vet* in future. Some practices are stagnating, others are going backwards, and many are selling out to corporate practices because they can no longer compete, but John has the bit between his teeth and is developing a practice that's going to be providing the type of service clients demand now and will still be suitable for the next twenty years.

I must admit that the main factor that drew me to Grace Lane was the fact that they still do farm work and moving there meant that I was introduced to several new characters, many of whom have appeared on *The Yorkshire Vet*, such as Abbie and her father Trevor, who have 450 dairy cows on their farm. Abbie is a remarkable woman and a true inspiration. She has dwarfism and so faces many challenges, which she overcomes. She has a fantastic and positive outlook on life and throws herself into the challenges of farming with great gusto.

One July at their farm I was called to do 'some' pregnancy diagnoses. The daybook said there were around forty cows to examine for pregnancy. It turned out to be ninety-seven! It was a logistical feat to get them all done, and they used their large circular milking parlour that holds fifty cows at a time. The first batch were all lined up ready for me when I arrived, with their bottoms presented. PDs are often done by feeling for changes in the uterus, which is accessed through the rectal wall. The stage of the pregnancy dictates what you feel. Under six weeks, for example, there is very little swelling in the uterus, but you can feel for the foetal membranes between your thumb and forefinger. It is an exacting technique that requires a lot of practice and nowadays is mainly carried out by ultrasound scanning. At eight weeks and over, the uterus becomes an elongated bag of fluid, and at about fourteen to sixteen weeks, structures develop in the uterus called cotyledons, which feel like corks bobbing about in water. Then later in pregnancy, when you get to about seven months, an artery develops in the uterus which is quite distinct. You can feel the vibrating woosh of blood running through this artery that supplements the blood supply to the uterus to nourish the calf during the later stages of pregnancy.

Fortunately, most of Trevor's were six to seven months in calf with just one or two not in calf at all, so they were fairly easy to check. There were only one or two in the early stages of pregnancy. Nevertheless, it was hard work. A cow's anal sphincter can be quite tight and so I had to force my arm in and then reach around inside with significant pressure applied by the anal muscles on my upper forearm, which started to feel bruised as time went on. In fact, by the end of ninety-seven cows' bottoms, the pain was quite considerable. Ten days later I still felt pain in my arm and thought to myself, this has got to be age related.

My work at Grace Lane also allowed me to meet new farming characters such as Andy Forbert. He is one of a dying breed of hill farmers. Viewers will have seen him on the TV show, and his dialect is so strong the producers of *The Yorkshire Vet* considered adding subtitles. I was quite proud of the fact that I understood every word he said and could happily join in with his banter. He lives in Farndale, has a very shrewd mind, and enjoys a laugh. One young chap, Luke, takes his sheep dogs around the farms and rounds up sheep for the farmers when needed. In the early stages of his shepherding career, Luke went to Andy's to help him round his sheep up off the hillsides. As the sheep neared the farm, being expertly marshalled by Luke and his dogs, Andy directed Luke to stand in a gap in the wall to stop the sheep escaping through it.

Andy instructed Luke to do so by saying: 'Go and stand in that gap and make a sound like a five-bar gate.' This type of humour is typical of the hardworking men of the Moors. When you get to know them well, they are the salt of the earth.

Andy likes a beer and has an arrangement with the landlady at his local pub. Customers who are looking for somewhere to pitch a tent are allowed to do so on his land. In exchange for him looking after her customers in this way, the landlady gives him a pint. Rumour has it, his tally got up to a hundred pints at one point. Apparently, he had them polished off in a week.

Luke, the shepherd, became another face on *The Yorkshire Vet*. His three-dog team is incredible. It consists of a mother, son and another, and they all work together as a team, guided by Luke's sometimes almost imperceptible commands. When those border collies are out in the field working, you can see that rounding up sheep is in their blood. It is exactly what they were born to do. Their levels of discipline, understanding of what's required, and concentration are phenomenal. Pip (my grandfather's boss's wayward canine) could have learned a lot from them.

A while ago one of the dogs, Badger, jumped off the quad bike and smashed his tibia and fibula into numerous fragments. Being such a horrible break it needed extensive surgery, which John and I performed. The bones needed to be realigned and fixed with plates and screws. The operation was filmed for the TV show.

To begin with, the recovery didn't go well, and for some reason that we didn't understand, Badger started having seizures. John got quite depressed about it, and worried that the dog was not going to recover, which is typical of colleagues in the profession who become attached to their patients. Even six weeks later, when I asked how the dog was doing, John would shake his head and say things were not looking good. 'He's still having seizures and he's not using the leg at all,' he said. 'I've told Luke to confine him. Rest him to give this thing a chance to heal. I just don't think Badger's going to make it.' The downbeat tone in John's voice was one of personal failure.

We didn't hear anything for some time from Luke until Jacob, our producer director on *The Yorkshire Vet*, decided to follow up the case and rang Luke to ask how Badger was getting on. To our delight, Badger had turned a corner and was doing really well. He was seemingly making a miraculous recovery. We decided to go and meet them and film a follow-up. I was fascinated to discover what had led to Badger's remarkable turnaround.

'What is it that's transformed Badger?' I asked Luke. 'We thought the chances of a recovery were slipping by.'

'I rested him and rested him, but he just continued carrying his leg and I knew I had to try something different,' explained Luke. 'So I took him out to see the sheep. All of a sudden, he went into work mode.'

At the sight of the sheep, something switched on in Badger's brain, and he went hell-for-leather with his mother and his mate to round up a group of sheep. From that day on, he's had no more seizures, and has never looked back.

It was a truly amazing and uplifting story. We filmed Badger back at work and took the footage back to show John at Grace Lane. He was so pleased he had tears in his eyes watching it. He couldn't believe what he was seeing. It is these emotions that patients such as Badger evoke in us.

Thankfully, injuries like that suffered by Badger are not seen on a daily basis. When it comes to dogs, possibly the most common complaint as vets we are confronted with is itchy skins, and it has become more common over the years.

There are so many conditions that we never get to the bottom of, such as allergies. The causes are often multifactorial and we often never get a clear picture of what causes them. They remain a puzzle and some cases are never solved. Sue Green, the boxer breeder, brought one of her bitches, Harriet, to see me at Skeldale because she had developed an urticarial reaction, which is an allergic skin reaction caused by histamine release in response to contact with an allergen in the food or the environment. You often see facial swelling, and in short-haired dogs like boxers, the hair stands up on the body forming what looks like a comical cobbled street appearance. More rarely in dogs, these reactions can be as serious or life-threatening as allergic reactions can be in humans.

The problem was quickly settled down with a steroid injection, but two weeks later Sue was back again with Harriet.

'It's happened again. I don't know what caused it,' she said, 'but it was very strange. Harriet was in the house, she went to the back door, and all she did was stand just outside. Suddenly these reactions started again. Can you tell me why, Mr Vet?' She asked with a 'gotcha' look on her face. I had no answers. It never happened again to Harriet and had to be put down to another of life's mysteries.

One of my earliest memories of strange animal behaviour was the case of Rex, who was one of our family dogs when I was a child. Rex was a lovely, gentle ex-gun dog who didn't enjoy the work he was tasked to carry out. Rex lived in an outside kennel. It was a small, old-fashioned raised chicken house on wheels. He was very comfortable and happy in there. He also came into the house, where he was equally relaxed. He was a happy dog who enjoyed his life following his premature retirement from the gun dog work which he hated. He'd be let out of his kennel in the mornings and go belting around, tail wagging, and then looking for breakfast before spending the majority of his time strolling around our land exploring any changes or new scents that he came across. But as he approached old age, his personality started to change. He became restless and wouldn't settle at night. He started to chew the wooden door and floor of the coop that had been his home all his life. Dad had to nail metal sheets on the inside of the door to stop him from destroying his house, which was totally out of character. Instead of relaxing and sleeping at night as he had always done, Rex spent all night ripping the sheets and nails out of his home. His personality change was something we couldn't comprehend. We left him in the house one day when we went out for a couple of hours, as we often did, and we returned to a badly gnawed window ledge and the curtains ripped from their rail and lying on the floor in tatters. He also started to defecate regularly in the house. It was a complete change of character, from being that of a happy, contented dog to one so distressed and confused.

Rex's character change was a puzzle but nowadays we commonly see animals showing behavioural changes as they age. I personally believe these changes in character are down to some form of dementia. It is becoming more common, I believe, because pets are living longer thanks to advances in care and nutrition. When I first qualified, if a cat reached fifteen years of age it had achieved a good age. Now, it's not uncommon for them to live to eighteen years and older. One day during consultations at Skeldale I had a twenty-year-old cat brought in to see me for a routine check-up and annual vaccinations. For her age she was remarkably fit. When I commented what a fantastic age she was, the owner explained that she had left the cat's mother at home strolling round the garden!

Another increasingly common condition we see in our pets, resulting from our lifestyle changes, is obesity and diabetes. We don't take as much exercise as we used to do, so dogs don't get as much exercise either. There are also a lot more treats available and people mollycoddle their pets much more than they used to. I see pets treated like children and dressed in outfits. They are sometimes seen as fashion accessories and status symbols. People don't realise that dressing an animal up is often distressing for the animal and could, in some cases, be construed as an act of cruelty.

Covid was a double-edged sword. In one way it reinforced our bonds with our pets. We had time to reflect on our busy lives. It afforded us time with them and perhaps we learned to appreciate them more. But it also created a massive demand for puppies, with sales going through the roof and prices rising to ridiculous levels. Consequently, unscrupulous puppy farmers stepped in to quench the market, because genuine bona fide breeders were unable to keep pace with demand.

As I watched all this unfold, I thought to myself: *This is only going to end in disaster when people have to go back to work*. And of course, it happened. Shelters and rehoming centres soon started to become overwhelmed with unwanted 'pandemic puppies' which had grown into adults. In some cases, owners no longer had the time to devote to their lockdown dogs. Dare I say it, for some, the novelty value just wore off, particularly for those who had taken on their dogs because of ill-conceived whims. Sadly, we live in a throwaway society where everything is disposable, even our pets, it would seem.

The pandemic-puppy rush also created a demand for so-called designer breeds such as the cavapoos and labradoodles, which were changing hands for several thousands of pounds. The irony is that they have fancy names and sell at a premium, but they're not pedigree breeds, they are cross breeds, what we used to call mongrels. But because they've got fancy names they sell for a premium.

The other sad trend I've seen become prevalent is how much pet sales are now influenced by fashion and celebrity status. If a certain influencer or reality star has a French bulldog, everybody wants one. And it seems to be these brachycephalic breeds that have become amongst the most fashionable; these are breeds such as bulldogs and pugs that can't breathe properly due to the fact that they have elongated soft palates, restricted airways and narrow nostrils. These dogs look cute, admittedly. And people think the gurgling noises they make are endearing. No, they're not. They are animals that are struggling to breathe.

I'm quite aware that all this makes me sound like a curmudgeon, and sometimes I am, but vets have a duty to animals, not just in the practice but in wider society, and maybe things have gone too far, and we need to reset our relationship with our animals. They are not toys, accessories or disposable playthings. We need to recognise them for the sentient creatures they are and treat them with respect. This includes breeding for better health and not pampering to the whims of the public who have been influenced to buy a certain breed because their favourite TV personality or pop star owns one.

I'll get off my soapbox now and finish where we started, with a couple of stories about Yorkshire farms and Yorkshire farmers.

Returning to Thirsk as a vet was a challenge, as many of the clients already knew me, and to my mind this familiarity brought with it greater expectations to succeed. One such client and, dare I say, distant family relative farmed in a picturesque village nestling at the foot of the Hambleton Hills. His name was Dick and he loved it when a bit of village gossip came his way. He revelled in it. The more depressing the news, the better as far as Dick was concerned.

This unhealthy preoccupation with bad news put a real spring in Dick's step. Once he'd offloaded it to someone, he went off on his way to spread his tales of woe to the next villager who crossed his path. This interest in bad news was only surpassed by his pessimism in the abilities of a vet delivering live lambs when called to help one of his ewes having problems at lambing time. In the office I witnessed many occasions when Dick called for help. One day it was my turn to go.

'I have a ewe to lamb. Can you get someone here quick?' he demanded.

'I'll get someone out as soon as possible, Dick,' the receptionist answered.

'As soon as possible! What does that mean? Whoever comes, tell 'em lambs will be dead afore he gets here.' And with that the phone would go dead.

I set off at a pace that could only be surpassed by Alladin on his magic carpet. On approaching the village, Dick was at the road junction to the farm. At the sight of my car, he started waving his hands frantically, looking like a possessed policeman on traffic duty.

With no pleasantries exchanged, his first words were: 'I doubt you'll be owr late.'

On entering the lambing shed I was greeted by an elderly lady standing watch over the ewe whose level of pessimism, incredibly, was even greater than Dick's. She was his neighbour, Cath.

'D' you think they'll be dead, Dick?' she enquired, cranking the level of fatalism up to the next level.

'Bound to be by now,' came Dick's inevitable reply.

On examining the contents of the ewe's reproductive tract under Dick and Cath's intense scrutiny, there was a palpable tension in the air. Within two minutes I delivered one of two lambs onto the deep straw bedding. It gasped as it gulped in the therapeutic Yorkshire air.

Cath broke the silence.

'Well, that beats hen racing, Dick,' she said. 'I wor sure it'd be dead but it looks as if it's alive. It must be a miracle.'

Soon after, the second lamb was born, breathing normally and sitting up, much to the amazement of Cath. Dick remained with a dignified and, I could tell, grateful silence.

As I drove away, I couldn't help smiling at the happy ending which had deprived Dick of another doom-and-gloom story to pass on during his village travels. It made me determined to deprive him still further on subsequent visits.

But perhaps one of my favourite stories, and a fitting one to end this book, involves Albert Noddins. He was typical in many ways of the clients I regularly met when I first qualified as a vet. He always looked at us vets a bit suspiciously. He wanted our help but didn't want to pay for it. In his view, vets were out purely to 'separate him from his hard earned brass' (money). This was the philosophy of many of these lads who would look sideways at us with suspicion and watch us with some degree of scepticism when we were really only trying to save their animals. One Saturday in my early career in Thirsk, Albert called Kirkgate to report that he had a litter of poorly piglets that were starting to die.

Albert wanted a chat first because if he could get some medicine for the piglets and save a visit, all the better.

I was on duty and answered the call.

Albert explained what the problem was and asked what he should be giving his piglets and how he should treat them.

'I think it might be better if I come and have a look, Mr Noddins,' I said.

'Alright vitnary, come and have a look if you think it's necessary or worth it,' he said, sighing. I knew what was going through his mind. He was doing a traditional Yorkshire calculation in his head, totting up what the piglets might be worth if cured and comparing that to the cost of treating them and, God forbid, the cost of the loss if the whole litter died.

I arrived in good time and went into the brick stable where his sows were kept when they gave birth. He ushered me over to the patients. There was a sow in a farrowing crate, which is a metal tubular construction to prevent the sows lying on the piglets when they are first born. She had twelve piglets, which was a good-sized litter. They looked in a very sorry state. Two had died already. Some of them were clinging on to life, hunched together, shivering and very weak. Their breathing was fast and shallow. My first thoughts were that they were too far gone to be saved. It was highly likely they were all going to die, I told myself.

'I won't lie to you, Mr Noddins,' I said, trying to give him some hope. 'They are in a bad way, and they may not make it. They are almost certainly suffering from a severe E. coli septicaemia. The prognosis is poor. In a lot of cases it will wipe out an entire litter.'

'Thought as much,' he replied.

I could almost read his mind. The look on his face said what a waste of time it was calling me out.

I treated them with what I thought would be the most effective antibiotic.

'Might be an idea if I could have a look in tomorrow,' I said.

Mr Noddins, having been given the grim prognosis, did the calculations in his head again.

'I don't know whether it's worth it, do you?' he said, again totting up the cost of a dead litter and not one, but two vet visits.

'I think it'd be a good idea if I bobbed my head in,' I pushed.

He fidgeted around, took his flat cap off, and scratched his head before rubbing his chin. His mind was in turmoil.

'Look, Mr Noddins, I'll do it free of charge,' I said, knowing that would be a game changer. 'I'll just charge you for the medication if there are any left to treat.'

'Aye, alright then,' he said resignedly.

I left fearing the worst and returned the following morning, Sunday at 10am, expecting to find a pile of dead bodies.

I had already made a few calls and was passing anyway, so it was not a problem to drop in and offer some words of condolence to Albert. I pulled up in the yard and called for him but he was not around, so I walked over to the outbuilding housing the sow and her babies.

I couldn't believe what I witnessed. The sow was lying contently, snoozing in the crate with the heat lamp on above her. She was surrounded by piglets, running about, squealing, and suckling well. I counted them. There were ten. We hadn't lost a single one.

As I was saying my silent prayers of joy, Mr Noddins appeared.

'Now then, Mr Noddins,' I offered as a well-used Yorkshire greeting. 'It's a bloody miracle; they're all still alive. Look at 'em.'

I felt jubilant at that moment. I felt like the best vet in the world. 'Successes like this should be celebrated,' I said.

Mr Noddins nodded his head then leaned forward, rested his arm on the low wall and looked at his piglets with a slight frown.

'Aye, they're doing alright maybe,' he conceded with a sigh. 'Not one's dead, alright.' Then he narrowed his eyes.

'Mind, you know, they've lost a bit of ground, haven't they?'

In other words, he was disappointed because they weren't in quite as good condition as if they hadn't had any infection.

I told Alf Wight that story the following day in the practice and I thought he'd never stop laughing.

'By, hell. You can't win,' he said as he chuckled. 'You'll never impress a Yorkshire farmer.'

But you can win, because tales like this, and the case of Badger the sheepdog, illustrate why we vets do what we do. I might moan sometimes, and look with wistful nostalgia at days gone by, but where else can you witness miracles on a regular basis, surrounded by some of the nicest people while caring for wonderful animals in a beautiful part of the world that I am lucky enough to call home?

Acknowledgments

Many thanks to Nick Harding, who spent many hours listening to me recall memories of my life and work as a veterinary surgeon and transformed them into readable prose.

Thank you also to Fritha Saunders and Mel Sambells at Mardle Books for all their help and advice.

A big thank you to Daisybeck Studios for allowing me to use some of their photographs taken during the course of my work when filming for *The Yorkshire Vet*, particularly Paul Stead (Chief Executive) and Mike Sinclair (Series Editor).

Thank you also to Amanda Stocks of Exclusive Press and Publicity who advises me on all publicity, media and promotional work, of which my knowledge is scant.

Thank you also to White Rose Books in Thirsk who champion the sales of my books far and wide.

Finally, I would like to thank my brother, David, who has aided and prompted when my memory has been a little sketchy.